French Chic

French Chic

40 Essentials an Elegant Parisian Woman Owns

Laura Merano

Coquilla Dorée

The image on the cover:

Insspirito

Pixabay.com

coquilledoree@gmail.com

ISBN: 978-83-971997-5-0

It's not the appearance, it's the essence.

It's not the money, it's the education.

It's not the clothes, it's the class.

Coco Chanel

Table of Contents

Introduction

French chic is a phenomenon revered worldwide, embodying timeless elegance and sophistication that has captivated fashion enthusiasts. In "French Chic: 40 Essentials an Elegant Parisian Woman Owns," we journey into the heart of Parisian elegance and style. This book serves as your passport to understanding and embracing the allure that French women effortlessly exude.

As the author, I had the privilege of engaging with ten Parisian women aged 22 and 73, each offering unique insights into French chic. They shared their perspectives, shaped by diverse life experiences. Their invaluable advice makes this book a comprehensive guide to achieving Parisian elegance. Through these intimate exchanges, I've curated a list of 40 essential items that every elegant Parisian woman embraces.

This journey into the world of French classic chic begins with exploring its origins, tracing its evolution from the court of Marie Antoinette to today's fashion houses. We delve into why Paris remains a global fashion hub, uncovering its enduring allure and secrets. The streets of this beautiful city serve as a runway, showcasing a unique blend of casual sophistication and charm that epitomizes French fashion. We explore the essential elements of French chic and reveal the daily rituals that keep Parisian style polished.

Learn how to adapt your wardrobe for every season and explore the vibrant palette of French chic. Discover how Parisian women dress for diverse occasions, from casual coffee dates to glamorous soirées, and gain inspiration from their philosophies on style and elegance. Practical tips from Parisian women will empower you to cultivate French chic, embracing elegance and confidence wherever you go.

Join me on this enchanting journey and discover how to infuse your life with the sophistication that defines Parisian women.

Laura Merano

I.

The History of French Chic Style

In the bustling streets of Paris, amidst the timeless architecture and lively cafes, Parisian women effortlessly embody a sense of style that has captivated the world for generations. Their approach to fashion goes beyond trends, representing a way of life rooted in elegance, individuality, and a deep appreciation for quality. French Chic, or "Parisian chic," is more than just a fashion statement – it reflects cultural heritage and personal expression. Each era of French fashion has contributed to the evolution of this iconic style, blending historical influences with modern sensibilities.

Beginnings and Early Inspirations

The French Chic style has its roots in the 18th century when France became the fashion capital of Europe. The French aristocracy, led by Marie

Antoinette, introduced new trends and extravagant outfits admired across the continent. Marie Antoinette, known for her love of luxurious fabrics and elaborate hairstyles, became a fashion icon of her time. Dresses with wide skirts, richly decorated with embroidery and lace, were symbols of prestige and elegance. Her hairstylist, Léonard Autié, was a pioneer in creating intricate hairstyles that became the hallmark of that era.

19th Century: The Birth of Modern Elegance

In the 19th century, during the reign of Napoleon III, Paris solidified its position as the world's fashion capital. Fashion houses like Worth began defining elegance through the introduction of haute couture. Charles Frederick Worth, considered the father of haute couture, introduced the concept of seasonal collections and individual fittings, attracting elites from around the world to Paris. The French style began to stand out for its simplicity of cut and attention to detail, which became the foundation of French Chic. Worth, known as the "architect of dresses," was the first to sign his creations, a revolutionary practice at the time.

Early 20th Century: The Revolution of Paul Poiret, Coco Chanel, and Madeleine Vionnet

One of the first designers to break away from the restrictive fashion of the past was Paul Poiret. In the early 20th century, Poiret abandoned corsets in favor of looser, more relaxed cuts, often drawing inspiration from oriental designs – his vibrant colors and luxurious fabrics diversified French fashion. Poiret was also a pioneer in organizing spectacular fashion shows that attracted media and public attention.

Another significant moment in the history of French Chic was the revolution brought by Coco Chanel. Chanel revolutionized fashion by introducing simple, elegant cuts and functional materials like jersey. Her designs, such as the little black dress and tweed suit, became style icons. Chanel promoted the idea that fashion should be comfortable yet elegant, perfectly aligning with the concept of French Chic.

Madeleine Vionnet, another prominent designer of this period, made significant contributions to the style with her innovative bias cut, giving garments fluidity and elegance that became the foundation of modern fashion. Vionnet revolutionized the way fabrics draped over the body, creating designs that were both comfortable and graceful.

1940s and 1950s: The Era of Lucien Lelong and Dior's New Look

During World War II, Lucien Lelong was crucial in maintaining the French fashion industry. His elegant and classic designs continue to inspire contemporary designers. As the chairman of the Chambre Syndicale de la Couture Parisienne, Lelong fought to protect French fashion houses during the German occupation.

After the war, Christian Dior introduced the "New Look" in 1947, revolutionizing fashion with a silhouette that featured a narrow waist, wide skirts, and emphasized bust. Dior restored femininity to fashion, contrasting with the practical and economical designs of the war years. His style represented the essence of post-war renewal and luxury, further cementing Paris's status as the fashion capital.

1950s and 1960s: Icons of Modern Style and André Courrèges

In the 1950s and 1960s, icons such as Brigitte Bardot and Audrey Hepburn became synonymous with Parisian chic. Bardot introduced elements of freedom and nonchalance into fashion, key aspects of French Chic. Her style was characterized by loose hairstyles, simple dresses, and flat shoes. Hepburn, although not French, was closely associated with Parisian fashion through her collaboration with designer Hubert de Givenchy. His designs for Hepburn, such as the little black dress from "Breakfast at Tiffany's," became fashion icons.

During this era, André Courrèges emerged as a pivotal figure in fashion. Known for his futuristic and avant-garde designs, Courrèges introduced the miniskirt and go-go boots, which became emblematic of the 1960s. His innovative use of materials like vinyl and his penchant for bright, bold colors influenced the fashion world significantly.

The History of French Chic Style

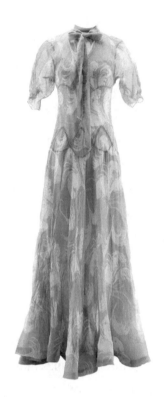

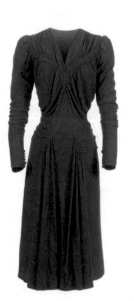

Classic French Chic from the second half of the 1930s, exemplified by dresses from the fashion houses of Madeleine Vionnet (top), Jeanne Paquin (left) and Jeanne Lanvin (right).

The History of French Chic Style

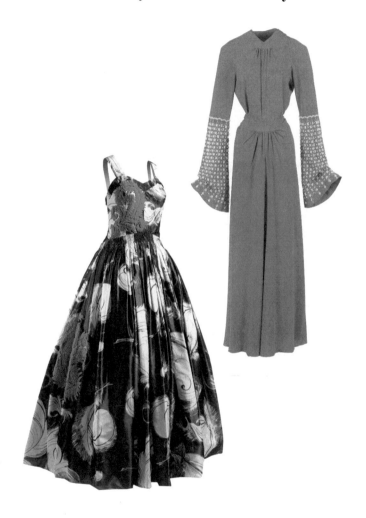

The History of French Chic Style

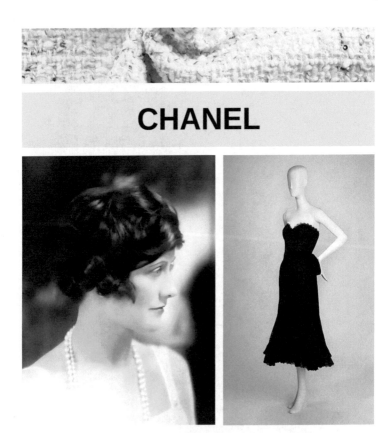

Coco Chanel had a significant influence on shaping French Chic. The legendary designer's clothing style is characterized by modesty and comfort. In the portrait, Coco Chanel in the 1920s.

The History of French Chic Style

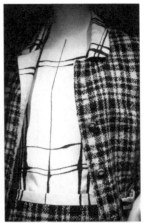

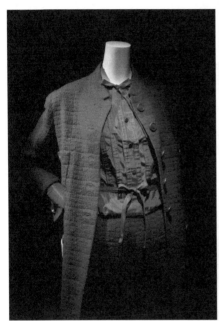

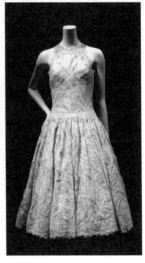

The History of French Chic Style

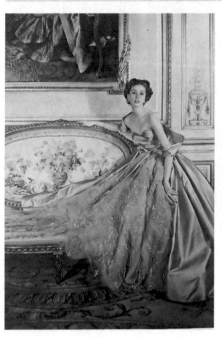

CHRISTIAN DIOR
PARIS

Abundant gathers, wide dress skirts, and many meters of fabric – these are the legendary creations of Dior. In the photo on the bottom left, the American model and actress Suzy Parker showcases the purple gown of the designer from 1953.

The History of French Chic Style

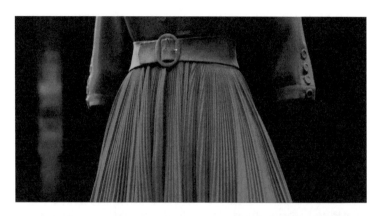

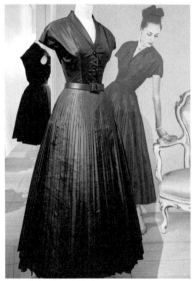

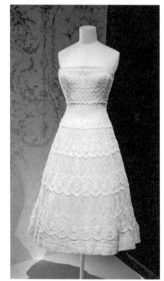

The Role of Fashion Designers
in the Development of French Chic

Pierre Balmain, another influential designer, was known for his refined elegance and ornate yet always stylish creations. His fashion house became a symbol of luxury and French chic. Balmain once said, "Elegance is the true beauty that never goes out of style."

Pierre Cardin became famous for his futuristic designs and innovative approaches to fashion. His bold and avant-garde creations, often inspired by space, influenced the development of French fashion and became an inspiration for many generations.

1970s and 1980s: Minimalism and Unisex

In the 1970s and 1980s, French designers like Yves Saint Laurent continued the tradition of elegance and simplicity. Saint Laurent introduced the tuxedo for women, a symbol of unisex fashion and emancipation. Minimalist cuts and neutral colors became the basis of French Chic. His designs combined elegance with functionality, which was revolutionary at the time.

Contemporary: Legacy and Modern Interpretations

Today, the French Chic style is not only continued but also reinterpreted by contemporary fashion icons such as Inès de La Fressange, Caroline de Maigret, and Jeanne Damas. This style still relies on simplicity, quality, and elegance. Modern interpretations often combine classic elements with contemporary trends, maintaining the spirit of effortless elegance. The French Chic style remains one of the most influential and desirable in the world, symbolizing timeless class and sophistication.

The History of French Chic Style

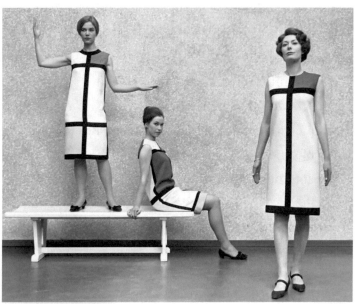

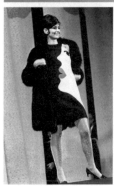

Yves Saint Laurent is another designer who contributed to establishing the French Chic style in the consciousness of fashion enthusiasts. Here are Laurents creations from 1966. At the top are the famous Mondrian dresses inspired by the works of Piet Mondrian.

The History of French Chic Style

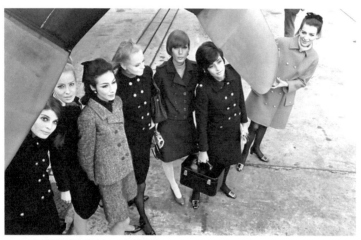

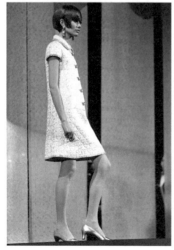
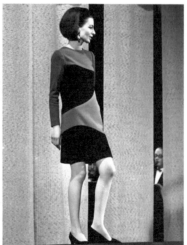

II.

Why Paris is the Fashion Capital

Paris, often hailed as the epicenter of global fashion, has an unparalleled reputation for its blend of history, innovation, and timeless elegance. The city's influence on fashion is deeply rooted in its culture, institutions, and the iconic designers who have called it home. Let's explore the reasons why Paris stands out as the fashion capital.

Education and Fashion Industry

Paris is home to several prestigious fashion schools, such as École de la Chambre Syndicale de la Couture Parisienne and Institut Français de la Mode. These institutions are renowned for rigorous training programs, producing future generations of top designers. Graduates from these schools include fashion icons like Yves Saint Laurent and Valentino Garavani, who have significantly shaped the industry.

Paris Fashion Week is one of the most crucial events in the fashion calendar, drawing designers, models, journalists, and buyers from around the globe. Held twice a year, this event showcases the latest collections from both established and emerging designers. It's a crucial platform for setting trends and dictating the future direction of global fashion. The origins of Paris Fashion Week can be traced back to 1945 when it began as an exclusive showcase for the world's elite.

Paris is the headquarters for many prestigious fashion houses, including Chanel, Dior, Givenchy, Yves Saint Laurent, and Hermès. These brands have played a pivotal role in shaping global trends.

Chanel's introduction of the "little black dress" and Dior's "New Look" are just a few examples of how Parisian designers have revolutionized fashion. Interestingly, the oldest French fashion house, Hermès, started in 1837 as a harness workshop before evolving into a symbol of luxury and style.

Culture and Lifestyle

Paris has always been a cultural hub where fashion, art, and literature intertwine. The city's cafes, theaters, galleries, and museums provide endless inspiration for designers and artists. For instance, the surrealist movement in the 1920s, with artists like Salvador Dalí and writers like André Breton, heavily influenced the fashion scene, encouraging avant-garde designs and bold creativity.

Parisians are known for blending simplicity with elegance, influencing global perceptions of French style. This effortless chic is characterized by a preference for quality over quantity, timeless pieces, and a natural approach to beauty. The concept of "less is more" is deeply ingrained in Parisian fashion philosophy, a legacy of Coco Chanel's minimalist designs.

The architectural beauty of Paris, with landmarks like the Eiffel Tower, Notre Dame, and the Louvre, adds to its status as the fashion capital. The city's aesthetic appeal provides a perfect backdrop for fashion shows and photoshoots, further cementing its place in fashion. Paris's historical significance as the birthplace of haute couture during the mid-19th century has left a lasting legacy on the industry.

The Streets of Paris

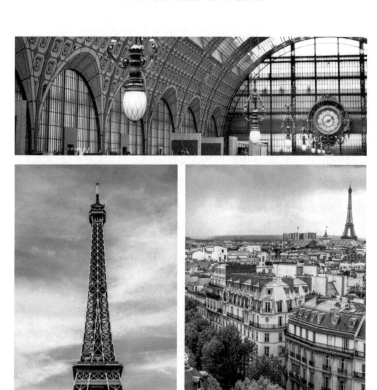

The Streets of Paris

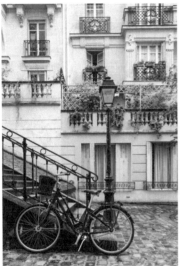
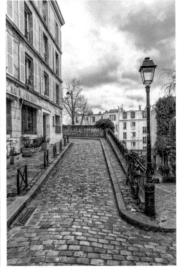

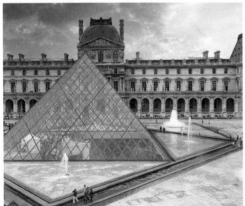

Paris continuously shapes and sets the global benchmarks for elegance and luxury. The city is a vibrant testament to fashion's legacy, trends, and future innovations.

A Legacy of Innovation and Influence

Paris, with its rich history, innovative designers, educational prowess, influential events, and unique culture, has earned its title as the world's fashion capital. The city continually inspires and defines global standards of elegance and luxury. From the cobblestone streets of Le Marais to the haute couture ateliers on Avenue Montaigne, Paris is a living, breathing embodiment of fashion's past, present, and future. The city's influence extends beyond clothing, impacting global beauty standards, lifestyle trends, and our perception of style and elegance.

III.

Elegant Life on the Streets of Paris

Paris, the City of Lights, is a place where daily life is infused with elegance and a vibrant, unspoken rhythm. The charm of Paris lies not only in its iconic landmarks but also in the everyday lives of its residents, who navigate the city with a distinctive flair.

Paris is a city where elegance and simplicity coexist beautifully. The daily lives of its residents are filled with cultural pursuits, stylish living, and a deep appreciation for the finer things. It is a place where history meets modernity, and each day offers new opportunities to experience the magic of this extraordinary city.

Streets Full of Life

The streets of Paris are always alive with activity. From early morning until late at night, there is a constant flow of people walking, cycling, and riding scooters. Parisians are known for their love of outdoor life. On weekends, parks like Jardin du Luxembourg, Parc des Buttes-Chaumont, and Jardin des Tuileries transform into lively hubs where families, friends, and couples gather. These green spaces are perfect for strolls, picnics, and outdoor activities such as yoga or jogging.

Cafés spill onto sidewalks, especially in vibrant neighborhoods like Le Marais, Saint-Germain-des-Prés, and Montmartre. Here, Parisians enjoy their morning coffee and croissants, catch up with friends over lunch, or indulge in an evening glass of wine while people-watching. The café culture is quintessentially Parisian, emphasizing the art of taking a moment to relax and observe the world.

The Parisian Style

Parisian fashion is synonymous with effortless elegance. Both men and women in Paris dress with a timeless sense of style that blends classic and contemporary elements. Neutral tones such as black, navy, gray, and beige dominate their wardrobes. Key pieces include well-tailored coats, chic blazers, and sophisticated scarves that elevate even the simplest of outfits.

Parisian women are often seen in midi dresses, tailored trousers, and understated skirts. Their accessories, from designer handbags to classic sunglasses and delicate jewelry, add a touch of refinement. Men in Paris opt for sharp suits, crisp shirts, and well-fitted trousers, always prioritizing quality over quantity. The emphasis on timeless pieces ensures that their wardrobes remain stylish for years.

Behavior and Etiquette

Parisians are known for their politeness and cultural sensitivity. Social interactions are marked by a certain formality, yet they remain warm and engaging. Greetings are a crucial aspect of Parisian etiquette – a friendly *bonjour* when entering shops or elevators is expected and appreciated. Among friends and close acquaintances, the customary kiss on the cheek, known as *la bise,* is a familiar greeting.

Life on the Streets of Paris

Parisian cafés spill onto the sidewalks, where locals enjoy morning coffee and croissants, catch up with friends over lunch, or indulge in an evening glass of wine while people-watching.

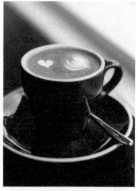

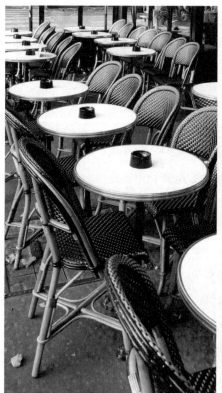

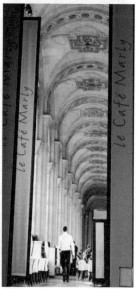

Life on the Streets of Paris

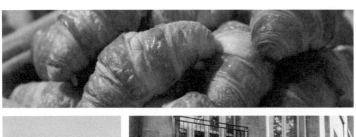

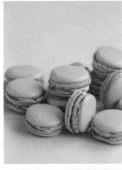

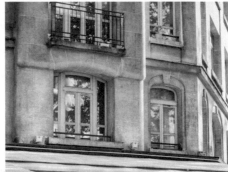

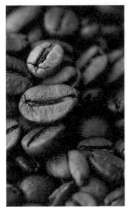

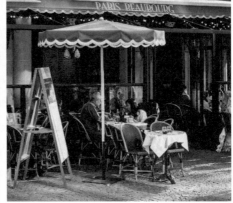

Dining out in Paris, whether at a cozy bistro or a Michelin-starred restaurant, involves a certain level of decorum. Parisians value good manners and respect for both staff and fellow diners. The pace of life slows down as meals become an opportunity to savor not just the food but the company and ambiance.

Leisure Activities

Parisians have a unique way of enjoying their leisure time. The city is a cultural treasure trove, and weekends are often spent exploring its many museums, galleries, and theaters. The Louvre, the Musée d'Orsay, and the Centre Pompidou are just a few of the world-renowned institutions that attract both locals and tourists alike.

Shopping is a beloved pastime in Paris. From haute couture boutiques on Rue Saint-Honoré to the eclectic vintage shops of Le Marais and the bustling antique markets like Marché aux Puces de Saint-Ouen, there is something for everyone. Parisians take pride in curating their wardrobes with pieces that are both stylish and enduring.

Evenings in Paris are magical. The bistros and wine bars come alive with the hum of conversation and the clink of glasses. Whether dining at a renowned Michelin-starred restaurant or a quaint local eatery, Parisians appreciate good food and fine wine. The Seine riverbanks, particularly near Île de la Cité and Île Saint-Louis, are popular spots for evening picnics and sunset watching, providing a romantic backdrop to the vibrant social life.

Daily Rituals

Life in Paris is marked by small, cherished rituals that add rhythm and joy to each day. A typical morning might start with a visit to a local boulangerie for fresh baguettes and croissants. Lunchtime often sees Parisians enjoying a leisurely meal at a nearby bistro or taking a stroll through one of the picturesque neighborhoods.

The markets, such as Marché d'Aligre and Marché des Enfants Rouges, are bustling with activity as locals shop for fresh produce, cheese, and other delicacies. These markets are not just places to buy food; they are social hubs where people connect and share in the culinary heritage.

IV.

Parisian Icons of Style, Talent, and Elegance

Paris, the city of lights, history, and timeless grace, has long attracted exceptional individuals who have become intertwined with its magical allure. Here are several remarkable women who have become icons of style, talent, and elegance, even though not all were born in the French capital.

These exceptional women, though diverse in origin, have captured hearts with their talent, personality, and dedication, leaving indelible marks on the history of culture, arts, and sciences. Their legacy inspires future generations, defining Paris as a place where talent meets extraordinariness.

Coco Chanel

Coco Chanel, a true fashion icon, was born into a humble family in France. However, she opened her first fashion boutiques in Paris that quickly became havens for elegant women worldwide. Chanel revolutionized haute couture with simple yet elegant designs, such as the little black dress and tweed suits. Her brand, Chanel, remains a symbol of luxury and taste untill today.

Brigitte Bardot

Brigitte Bardot, an icon of the 1960s, born in Paris, captured attention on screen and off with her wild, independent style and bombshell persona in French cinema. Bardot is also known for her advocacy for animal rights and environmental causes, adding depth to her inspiring character.

Juliette Binoche

Juliette Binoche, an Oscar-winning actress, was born in Paris and is one of the most talented actresses of her generation. Her career spans roles in art-house films and commercial successes, earning acclaim for emotional portrayals. Binoche also engages in charitable work and supports arts and culture, making her one of the most respected figures in French and international cinema.

Carla Bruni

Carla Bruni, a model, singer, and former First Lady of France, symbolizes elegance and style. Despite her Italian roots, her connection to Paris contributed to her musical career and role as an ambassador of French fashion and culture. Her dedication to charity work and promoting education makes her an inspiring and influential figure.

Édith Piaf

Édith Piaf, known as the "Little Sparrow" of French song, although born in Paris, led a life filled with drama and passion, making her songs resonate with listeners worldwide to this day. Her interpretations of classics like "La Vie en Rose" and "Non, je ne regrette rien" have immortalized her in French musical culture.

Simone de Beauvoir

Simone de Beauvoir, a philosopher, writer, and feminist icon, was born in Paris and spent life deeply involved in the city's intellectual life. Her book "The Second Sex" had a profound impact on the global women's emancipation movement, challenging traditional gender roles and advocating for equality. Beauvoir continues to inspire generations of women striving for autonomy and equality.

Marie Curie

Marie Curie, born in Poland but closely associated with France throughout her life, is one of the most renowned female scientists in history. A two-time Nobel Prize laureate in physics and chemistry for her pioneering research on radioactivity, Curie was not only a brilliant scientist but also a symbol of intellectual strength and determination. Her legacy is carried on by scientific institutions worldwide.

Marion Cotillard

Marion Cotillard, a French actress, and Oscar winner for her role as Edith Piaf in "La Vie en Rose," is an artist of versatile talent and extraordinary charm. Her films have garnered acclaim in both Europe and Hollywood, and her ability to embody diverse roles makes her one of the most respected actresses of her generation.

Audrey Tautou

Audrey Tautou, known for her role in the iconic film "Amélie," embodies the delicacy and grace of French cinema. Born in Beaumont, her career includes roles in both art-house movies and commercial successes. Her charming personality and natural elegance make her one of the most recognizable faces of French cinema worldwide.

Inès de La Fressange

Inès de La Fressange, a model and style icon, was born in Gassin, France. Her refined taste and impeccable style have made her a role model in the fashion world and a symbol of French class and sophistication.

V.

French Chic Moments
in Film and Media

French Chic, with its timeless elegance and effortless style, has been immortalized in numerous films and media, shaping fashion trends and inspiring generations. These iconic moments not only highlight the allure of French fashion but also illustrate how cinema and media have played a pivotal role in popularizing and perpetuating the French Chic aesthetic.

Audrey Hepburn in
"Breakfast at Tiffany's" (1961)

While Audrey Hepburn was not French, her portrayal of Holly Golightly in "Breakfast at Tiffany's" featured a quintessentially French sense of style. The little black dress designed by Hubert de Givenchy became a global sensation, embodying the essence of French Chic. Hepburn's elegant updo, oversized sunglasses, and pearl necklace created a look that remains iconic today. Givenchy's collaboration with Hepburn set a precedent for the designer-actress relationship in Hollywood, blending French haute couture with cinematic glamour.

Brigitte Bardot in
"And God Created Woman" (1956)

Brigitte Bardot's role in "And God Created Woman" introduced her as an international sex symbol and a fashion icon. Her carefree, sultry style, characterized by tousled hair, form-fitting dresses, and ballet flats, epitomized the French Chic aesthetic of the 1950s. Bardot's influence extended beyond film, impacting global fashion with her signature off-the-shoulder tops and gingham prints. Her fashion choices in the film reflected the liberating spirit of post-war France, resonating with women who sought comfort and allure in their clothing.

Catherine Deneuve in "Belle de Jour" (1967)

Catherine Deneuve's portrayal of Séverine in "Belle de Jour" is another landmark in French cinema that showcases French Chic. Deneuve's sophisticated wardrobe, designed by Yves Saint Laurent, featured tailored coats, shift dresses, and chic accessories, reinforcing her image as the epitome of French elegance. His designs for "Belle de Jour" set trends for minimalist yet refined fashion, influencing both high fashion and everyday style.

Jane Birkin in "La Piscine" (1969)

Jane Birkin's effortless style in "La Piscine" captured the essence of French Chic in the late 1960s. Her casual yet stylish outfits, including the iconic white shirt and denim shorts, highlighted her natural beauty and relaxed approach to fashion. Birkin's ability to blend simplicity with sophistication has made her a perennial style icon. Her style in "La Piscine" exemplified the merging of British and French fashion influences, creating a unique and enduring look.

Icons of Style and Elegance

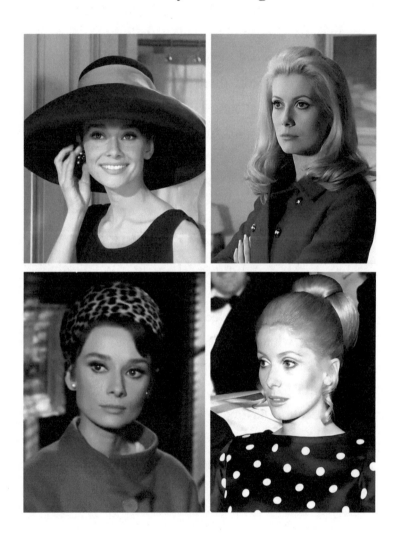

Icons of Style and Elegance

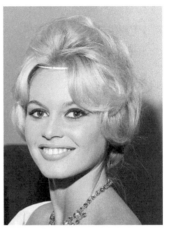

Catherine Deneuve, Audrey Hepburn, and Brigitte Bardot – icons of French Chic. These style legends embody the Parisian allure that blends classic beauty with modern flair.

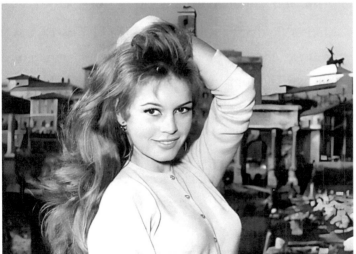

Anna Karina in Jean-Luc Godard's Films

Anna Karina's roles in Jean-Luc Godard's films, such as "Vivre sa Vie" (1962) and "Pierrot le Fou" (1965), encapsulate the French New Wave's impact on fashion. Her playful yet chic style, featuring mod dresses, striped tops, and bold accessories, captured the youthful, avant-garde spirit of 1960s France. Karina's fashion in Godard's films reflected the era's revolutionary approach to cinema and style, emphasizing individuality and artistic expression.

Marion Cotillard in "La Vie en Rose" (2007)

Marion Cotillard's portrayal of Édith Piaf in "La Vie en Rose" brought French Chic to the contemporary cinema. The film's costume design, inspired by the 1940s and 1950s, showcased elegant, vintage French fashion. Cotillard's performance and the film's visual style paid homage to Piaf's iconic looks, blending historical accuracy with cinematic artistry. The film's success reintroduced vintage French fashion to modern audiences, sparking a renewed interest in classic French styles.

Lea Seydoux in
"Blue is the Warmest Color" (2013)

Lea Seydoux's portrayal of Emma in "Blue is the Warmest Color" presented a modern interpretation of French Chic. Her character's distinctive, edgy style, featuring minimalist clothing and natural makeup, resonated with contemporary viewers. Seydoux's fashion choices in the film, including her iconic blue hair, reflected a blend of traditional French elegance and modern individuality. The film's raw and realistic depiction of relationships, coupled with Seydoux's fashion, highlighted the evolving nature of French Chic in the 21st century.

From the vintage elegance of Catherine Deneuve to the modern minimalism of Lea Seydoux, iconic moments in film and media have continuously shaped and redefined French Chic. These portrayals not only celebrate the timeless qualities of French fashion but also showcase its adaptability and enduring influence. Through cinema and media, French Chic remains a dynamic and inspirational force, encouraging individuality and timeless elegance.

VI.

Elements of French Chic

The allure of French Chic style is its effortless blend of elegance, simplicity, and timelessness. Rooted in the cultural and historical fabric of France, this style has been celebrated for its understated yet sophisticated approach to fashion. From the bustling streets of Paris to the picturesque countryside, French women have mastered the art of looking impeccably stylish without appearing to try too hard. This chapter delves into the key elements that define French Chic, revealing the secrets behind this enduring aesthetic.

Minimalism

One of the foundations of French Chic is minimalism, which involves choosing simple cuts and classic lines that never go out of style. The idea is to maintain an elegant yet understated wardrobe that is both stylish and practical.

Simple Cuts

French women often opt for clothing with simple lines that are easy to mix and match, always looking chic. Examples include plain white shirts, well-tailored blazers, and classic jeans. This simplicity allows for versatility and elegance in everyday outfits.

Classic Lines

Modern classic silhouettes help create a wardrobe that is timeless and versatile. This approach encourages investing in pieces that can be worn for many years, maintaining their appeal and functionality.

Quality

Investing in high-quality materials and clothing is another crucial element of French Chic. Quality fabrics not only look better but also retain their appearance longer, emphasizing the importance of durability and luxury.

High-Quality Fabrics

Materials like wool, silk, cashmere, and linen are commonly chosen by those who prefer French Chic.

These fabrics have a luxurious look and feel and are known for their longevity.

Attention to Detail

Clothes with meticulous finishing and precise stitching are essential. The quality of craftsmanship affects both the durability and the aesthetic appeal of the garments.

Effortless Elegance

French Chic is often associated with a look that appears effortless yet well-thought-out. It's about mastering the art of looking elegant without seeming to try too hard.

Casual Hairstyles

Natural-looking hair, often slightly tousled, is typical of French Chic. This style avoids elaborate hairstyles in favor of a relaxed, easygoing look.

Makeup

Subtle makeup that enhances natural beauty is another key element. French women often choose minimalist makeup with a focus on one feature, like a bold red lip, to maintain an elegant appearance.

Elements of French Chic

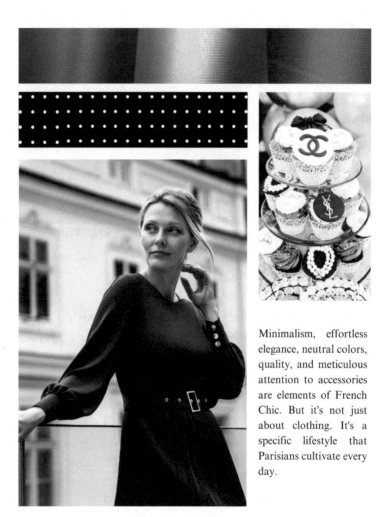

Minimalism, effortless elegance, neutral colors, quality, and meticulous attention to accessories are elements of French Chic. But it's not just about clothing. It's a specific lifestyle that Parisians cultivate every day.

Elements of French Chic

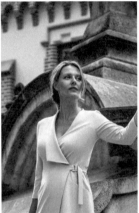

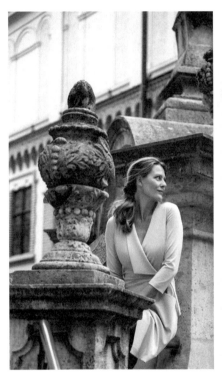

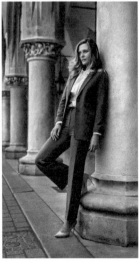

Neutral Colors

The color palette of French Chic consists mainly of neutral colors, which are easy to mix and match and always look sophisticated.

Black and White

These two colors are the cornerstone of any French wardrobe. Black is versatile and chic, while white adds freshness and lightness to outfits.

Greys and Beiges

These colors are perfect for creating subtle and refined ensembles. They can be easily paired with other neutrals or more vibrant accents, maintaining a balanced and elegant look.

Accessories

Accessories play a significant role in French Chic. They are carefully selected to complement an outfit without overwhelming it.

Jewelry

Delicate jewelry, such as gold or silver earrings and subtle necklaces, adds elegance without excess. The preference is for timeless pieces that enhance the overall look.

Scarves and Silk Scarves

These accessories are often used to add color and texture to simple outfits. French women frequently wear silk scarves, which can be tied in various ways to create different looks.

VII.

French Chic in the Daily Lives
of Parisians

The French Chic style profoundly shapes the everyday lives of elegant Parisians, influencing their approach to fashion, work, social relationships, and overall lifestyle. French Chic is more than just a fashion choice – it is a holistic lifestyle that combines elegance, simplicity, and an appreciation for quality in every aspect of life. This sophisticated approach ensures that French Chic remains a beloved and enduring style for women worldwide. Here is how this distinctive style permeates various aspects of their daily routines.

Wardrobe and Dressing

Effortless Mix and Match

Parisians are masters at creating chic outfits with minimal effort. They invest in versatile, high-quality pieces that can be effortlessly combined to create numerous looks. This ensures their wardrobes remain both stylish and practical.

Subtle Statements

Instead of chasing every trend, Parisians choose timeless pieces that make subtle yet impactful statements. A perfectly tailored blazer or a classic trench coat can elevate any outfit without appearing overly flashy.

Functional Elegance

Clothing that is both functional and elegant is a priority. Parisians favor items like well-fitted jeans, crisp white shirts, and comfortable yet stylish shoes that allow them to navigate their busy city lives with ease.

Lifestyle

Simplicity in Living

The French Chic lifestyle emphasizes simplicity and quality. Parisians favor a clutter-free environment, focusing on a few cherished items rather than an excess of possessions. This minimalist approach extends to their homes, where elegant yet functional decor creates a serene atmosphere.

Cultural Enrichment

Engaging in artistic activities is a significant part of Parisian life. Regular visits to museums, art galleries, and theaters provide continuous inspiration and intellectual stimulation.

Culinary Appreciation

Enjoying good food and wine is a key aspect of the French Chic lifestyle. Parisians take time to savor meals, whether at home or in their favorite bistros, appreciating the experience of dining well.

Work and Career

Effortless Professionalism

In their professional lives, Parisians blend elegance with ease. Their work attire is sophisticated yet comfortable, enabling them to move seamlessly from the office to social engagements. They favor tailored trousers, simple blouses, and classic dresses that exude professionalism without compromising on style.

Balanced Approach

Maintaining a healthy balance between work and personal life is crucial. Parisians value time spent with loved ones and engage in activities that nourish their well-being, ensuring that career ambitions do not overshadow personal happiness.

Social Relationships

Graceful Interactions

Social interactions are approached with the same elegance that defines their style. Politeness, respect, and charm are integral to daily conversations, whether with close friends or new acquaintances. This graciousness is a hallmark of the French Chic way of life.

Thoughtful Gatherings

Social gatherings are an essential part of Parisian life. Whether hosting intimate dinner parties or attending cultural events, Parisians place a high value on quality interactions and meaningful connections. These gatherings often reflect their refined tastes and deep love for sophisticated enjoyment.

Additional Insights

Historical Influence

French Chic is deeply rooted in the historical and cultural heritage of Paris. The city's legacy of influential designers and fashion icons continues to inspire new generations, providing a foundation for the timeless elegance that defines French Chic.

Global Inspiration

While firmly anchored in French culture, French Chic also draws inspiration from worldwide influences. Parisians are open to incorporating elements from other cultures, blending them seamlessly with their traditions to create a unique and dynamic style.

VIII.

40 Essentials of an Elegant Parisian Woman

Elegance is a hallmark of Parisian style, effortlessly blending timeless fashion with a touch of personal flair. To uncover the secrets behind this iconic elegance, I engaged in conversations with ten of my Parisian friends, all of whom are renowned for their impeccable style in any situation. These women graciously allowed me a look into their wardrobes and dressing tables, revealing the carefully curated items that define their chic looks.

From our conversations and my observations, I compiled a list of forty essential items that consistently appeared in their collections. This list reflects the foundational pieces that contribute to the elegance and sophistication synonymous with Parisian fashion. Whether it's a classic trench coat, a pair of stylish earrings, or a signature red lipstick, these essentials form the cornerstone of an elegant woman's wardrobe and beauty routine. Join me as we explore the timeless and versatile items that embody the essence of Parisian chic.

1. Silk Button-Up Blouse

A quintessential piece, the silk button-up blouse brings a touch of timeless elegance to any outfit. Available in pure white, off-white (écru), beige, or light peach, it elevates the formality of your look and highlights the uniqueness of any occasion. The subtle sheen of silk brightens the face, making this blouse a versatile and enduring addition to any wardrobe.

How to Wear

Pair with high-waisted trousers for a polished office look, or tuck into a pencil skirt for a chic dinner outfit. Layer under a classic blazer for added sophistication.

2. Smooth Turtleneck

This practical yet stylish item protects against the cold and adds a touch of casual sophistication. Knitted from lightweight yarns such as wool, silk, cotton, or viscose, it fits snugly around the neck and sits comfortably under a blazer. Available in monochrome hues and classic colors, it is perfect for layering and adds a refined touch.

How to Wear

Layer under a blazer or cardigan for a refined look. Pair with a pleated skirt for an elegant touch, or wear with jeans and ankle boots for a casual day out.

3. Linen Shirt

Ideal for summer, the linen shirt offers excellent protection against high temperatures and stylish wrinkles to add character. It effortlessly replaces a T-shirt – roll up the sleeves and unbutton the top two buttons. Available in solid colors like white, blue, turquoise, pale pink, and pastel yellow, or striped versions such as white-blue, white-navy, white-pink, or white-yellow, it ensures a cool and chic summer look.

How to Wear

Roll up the sleeves and wear with tailored shorts for a breezy summer outfit. Pair with a midi skirt for a relaxed yet chic look, or layer over a swimsuit at the beach.

4. Breton Striped T-Shirt

The Breton striped t-shirt, or marinière, infuses nautical charm and casual elegance into any outfit. Typically featuring horizontal navy and white stripes, this piece embodies effortless French style. Made from soft, breathable cotton, it offers comfort and versatility. With its classic boat neckline and three-quarter length sleeves, it pairs perfectly with pants, or a skirt.

How to Wear

Team with straight-leg jeans and ballet flats for a classic French look. Layer under a trench coat or blazer, or tuck into a pleated skirt for a playful twist.

5. Midi Skirt

A hallmark of classic elegance, the midi skirt is essential. Covering the knee and reaching mid-calf, it comes in flattering silhouettes such as pencil, trapezoidal, wrap-around, and circle-cut, with a godet or pleats. Made from flowing, noble fabrics, preferably lined, and featuring a buttoned waistband, it's available in darker shades of classic colors.

How to Wear

Style with a silk blouse and low-heeled court shoes for a refined office look. Pair with a turtleneck and boots for a cozy fall outfit, or a simple blouse for a casual day out.

6. Pleated Skirt

Nostalgic yet unpretentious and stylish, the pleated skirt, also known as a plissé skirt, drapes beautifully. It pairs well with a classic blazer and silk button-up blouse, as well as a turtleneck, cardigan, or sweater. Available in white for spring-summer or darker classic colors for fall-winter, it adds a retro touch to any outfit.

How to Wear

Pair with a classic blazer and silk blouse for a sophisticated ensemble. Combine with a sweater and ankle boots for a chic fall look, or a turtleneck and flats for effortless elegance.

French Chic in Everyday Outfits

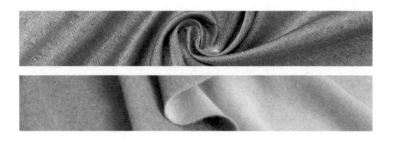

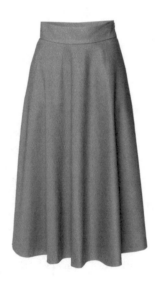
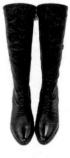

The midi skirt is a staple in the wardrobe of every elegant Parisian. It can be paired with a variety of accessories. A-line and gathered waist models made from luxurious, thicker fabrics look great with a turtleneck, pullover, blazer, and boots. Beige and camel colors complement gray and black beautifully.

French Chic in Everyday Outfits

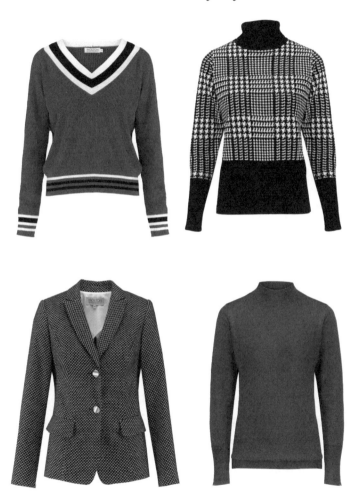

7. Fabric Pants

Indispensable for an elegant wardrobe, classic fabric pants create a look as sophisticated as a midi skirt. Made from well-draping fabric, they come in darker shades from the classic color palette. Typically featuring a belt, pockets, a regular or high waist, and a maxi length or just above the ankle, they are available in cigarette cuts or wide-leg styles, ensuring the fabric doesn't cling to the thighs.

How to Wear

Wear with a silk button-up blouse and loafers for a smart casual look. Pair with a turtleneck and blazer for a polished outfit, or a simple t-shirt and ballet flats for a relaxed day out.

8. Dark Wash Straight-Leg Jeans

A timeless classic, dark wash straight-leg jeans are a must-have. Crafted from high-quality denim, they offer a sleek and flattering fit. The dark indigo color is slimming and versatile, suitable for dressing up or down. Their practicality and enduring style make them a cornerstone of everyday elegance.

How to Wear

Pair with a silk blouse and ballet flats for a chic daytime look. Style with a tailored blazer and heels for a sophisticated evening ensemble, or a cotton sweater and sneakers for a casual outfit.

9. Chino Pants

Versatile and essential, chino pants bridge the gap between casual and semi-formal attire. Made from lightweight cotton twill, they offer comfort and durability. Featuring a mid-rise waist, straight-leg cut, and minimalistic design with concealed pockets and a flat front, they are available in classic shades like khaki, navy, and black.

How to Wear

Dress with a blazer and loafers for a smart casual look. Pair with a t-shirt and sneakers for a relaxed day out, or a button-up shirt and ballet flats for a polished outfit.

10. Smooth Cardigan

This button-up warmer adds a touch of ease to classic combinations. Paired with a silk button-up blouse or turtleneck, it is knitted from softly draping noble yarn. Featuring a buttoned front, round or V-neckline, narrower sleeves, and a length that reaches just below the hips, it's available in monochrome basic or complementary classic colors.

How to Wear

Layer over a silk blouse and trousers for a refined office look. Pair with a midi skirt and turtleneck for a cozy fall outfit, or wear with jeans and a t-shirt for a casual day out.

11. Cotton Sweater

A casual staple for the spring-summer season, the cotton sweater fits perfectly into any wardrobe. Thick-knitted with visible stitching (including cable knits), it's pulled over the head and features a round or V-neckline. Available in pure or off-white (écru) or navy blue, it can be monochrome or striped, reminiscent of sailor clothing, and protects against wind and cool summer evenings.

How to Wear

Pair with a pleated skirt and ballet flats for a chic spring outfit. Layer over a linen shirt and jeans for a relaxed look, or wear with chino pants and loafers for a casual yet polished ensemble.

12. Classic Blazer

A classic blazer adds strength and formality to any outfit. Featuring a traditional cut with waist shaping, a collar, slightly raised shoulders, button closure, and a length that reaches between the waist and hips, it is made from smooth, wrinkle-resistant, single-colored fabric in the dark (black, navy blue, brown) or light (ashen, beige) tones.

How to Wear

Wear over a silk blouse and fabric pants for a sophisticated office look. Pair with jeans and a turtleneck for a smart casual outfit, or layer over a dress for added formality.

13. Summer Jacket

Perfect for spring-summer outfits needing a touch of formality, the classic-length summer jacket is slightly tailored, and buttoned, with a collar and pockets. Made from breathable fabrics like cotton blends, it is available in light classic colors like white, écru, beige, and ash, as well as pastel shades of blue, pink, green, or yellow.

How to Wear

Layer over a linen shirt and chinos for a warm-weather look. Pair with a pleated skirt and cotton sweater for a chic spring outfit, or wear with a cocktail dress for added formality.

14. Cocktail Dress

An elegant cocktail dress is perfect for formal daytime events such as ceremonial dinners, business lunches, and afternoon receptions. This chic midi-length dress features understated tailoring and long or 3/4 sleeves and is available in darker shades from the classic color palette. Accessories can be adjusted to suit the occasion, enhancing its refined character.

How to Wear

Pair with low-heeled court shoes and a small classic handbag for a refined look. Accessorize with elegant jewelry for a formal event, or dress with a cardigan for a casual setting.

15. Little Black Dress

An iconic wardrobe staple, the little black dress embodies timeless elegance and simplicity. Designed to flatter any figure with its clean lines and classic cut, it typically features a fitted bodice and a hemline just above the knee. Made from high-quality fabrics like silk, crepe, or wool, it remains a durable and stylish choice in any wardrobe.

How to Wear

Style with a statement necklace and heels for an evening out. Pair with a blazer and flats for a chic office look, or accessorize with a silk scarf for a touch of elegance.

16. Classic Evening Gown

For formal occasions, a classic evening gown is indispensable. Featuring a fitted bodice and a flowing, floor-length skirt it is made from luxurious materials like silk, satin, or chiffon. Available in classic colors such as black, deep red, or navy blue, details like a sweetheart neckline, delicate lace overlay, or a subtle train enhance its elegance, making you feel like the epitome of grace and poise at any event.

How to Wear

Pair with elegant jewelry and heels for a formal event. Accessorize with a clutch and a silk scarf for added sophistication, or wear with a wool coat for a polished winter look.

17. Trench Coat

A timeless outerwear piece that exudes effortless sophistication and versatility, the trench coat is an indispensable part of a Parisian wardrobe. Typically crafted from water-resistant fabric like cotton gabardine, it features a double-breasted front, a belted waist, and a knee-length or longer cut. The classic beige or khaki color makes it suitable for both casual and formal occasions, while the epaulets, storm flaps, and cuff straps add distinctive style elements.

How to Wear

Throw over a silk blouse and fabric pants for a chic daytime look. Pair with jeans and a turtleneck for a casual outfit, or layer over a trouser suit for added elegance.

18. Wool Coat

An essential piece of the winter wardrobe for every elegant woman, no jacket from a renowned brand can replace it. This well-tailored coat, made from high-quality fabric with at least 80% wool, has been an investment for many years. With a classic tailored cut and midi length, it is lined and features slightly raised shoulders with the help of pads. This model has a traditional cut and timeless character, devoid of unnecessary decorations, and comes in light shades (beige, caramel, ash) or dark shades (black, graphite, brown, navy blue, burgundy) from the basic palette of classic colors.

How to Wear

Layer over a turtleneck and fabric pants for a sophisticated winter look. Pair with a midi skirt and boots for a cozy fall outfit, or wear with a cocktail dress for added formality.

French Chic in Everyday Outfits

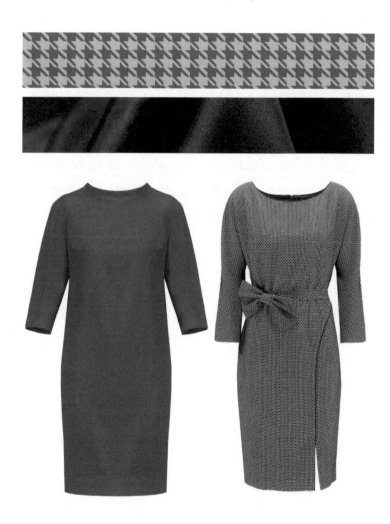

French Chic in Everyday Outfits

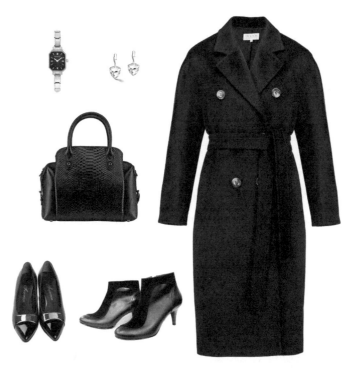

These two cocktail dresses are ideal for cooler days. Their timeless style makes them versatile for pairing with different accessories. They achieve a festive allure when adorned with bold jewelry and high-heeled pumps. A classic watch, ankle boots, and a spacious handbag lend them a casual appearance. These dresses should be worn with a coat as outerwear. Burgundy and gray harmonize beautifully with black and silver hues.

19. Headwear for a Coat

Formal outerwear calls for elegant headwear that a woolen cap cannot replace. A hat, pillbox, beret, or cloche hat complements the coat perfectly. Made of firm and smooth fabric (usually woolen), this headwear is stiffer than a loose-knit cap and may have decorations such as a brim, draped fabric appliqué, or a brooch, adding a refined touch to the overall look.

How to Wear

Pair a hat or beret with a wool coat for a classic winter look. Accessorize with a pillbox hat for formal occasions, or a cloche hat for a touch of vintage elegance.

20. Silk Scarf

A stylish essential for every elegant woman. Its pattern should complement the complexion, hair color, and the colors of favorite wardrobe items. Made of luxurious silk with hand-sewn edges, it may be second-hand from a vintage store or an online auction. It doesn't have to be from the latest collection of a famous brand, as lesser-known manufacturers offer equally beautiful high-quality scarves, making it a timeless accessory.

How to Wear

Tie around your neck for a classic look, or wear it as a headscarf for added elegance.

21. Straw Hat

Adds elegance to summer headwear. This hat is much more stylish than a canvas cap, baseball cap, or sporty visor. Made of natural straw rather than imitation woven paper, it is tailored to fit the face and silhouette. Available in classic colors: white or a light or dark shade of beige, it features a grosgrain ribbon encircling its crown, offering a chic and timeless summer accessory.

How to Wear

Pair with a linen shirt and shorts for a breezy summer look. Wear with a midi dress for added sophistication, or combine with a swimsuit for a chic beach outfit.

French Chic in Everyday Outfits

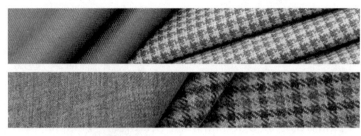

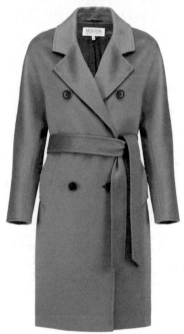

A classic wool coat is a must-have in the wardrobe of an elegant Parisian woman. It pairs beautifully with simple trousers, a plain turtleneck, and Chelsea boots. The shades of beige and brown blend perfectly with black.

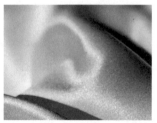

French Chic in Everyday Outfits

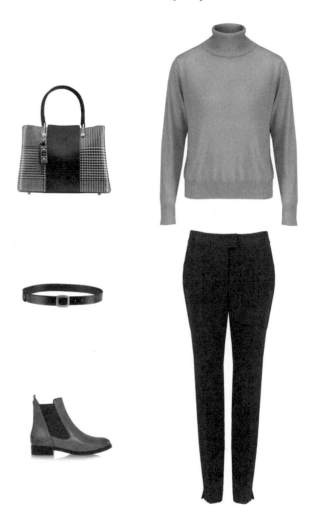

22. Leather Gloves

The accessory that elevates outerwear to a higher level of elegance. Unlike knit or fabric gloves, leather gloves emphasize the nobility of the attire and pair perfectly with a formal coat. Made of good quality, they are soft and may feature stitching or small embellishments (such as buttons). The autumn-winter version has a woolen fabric lining, while the spring model is made with thin leather or suede.

How to Wear

Pair with a wool coat for a polished winter look. Wear with a trench coat for added elegance, or accessorize with a classic handbag for a refined touch.

23. Woolen Scarf

A wardrobe essential for the autumn-winter season, this woolen scarf can be worn under or over a coat, or draped over the shoulders. A beautiful, densely woven, sizable woolen scarf also serves as a stylish addition to a jacket or dress made of thicker fabric. Patterned or plain, it complements the complexion, hair color, and the colors of favorite clothing items, adding warmth and elegance.

How to Wear

Drape over your shoulders for a cozy look. Pair with a wool coat for added warmth, or wear with a classic blazer for a chic fall outfit.

24. Classic Everyday Handbag

The classic everyday handbag is a practical yet stylish accessory, designed to complement any outfit while providing ample space for daily essentials. Crafted from high-quality leather, it often features a structured shape, sturdy handles, and a detachable shoulder strap for versatility. Colors like black, tan, or navy ensure the bag's versatility, making it suitable for casual and formal settings. The timeless design may include subtle hardware accents, such as gold or silver zippers and clasps, ensuring it remains a staple in your wardrobe for years.

How to Wear

Pair with a silk blouse and fabric pants for a polished office look. Wear with jeans and a cotton sweater for a casual outfit, or accessorize with a dress for added elegance.

25. Small Classic Handbag

A stylish element that complements an outfit with a light character, such as cocktail dresses, summer sets with trousers, and combinations of blouses and skirts. This small, lightweight handbag blends well with silk, chiffon, georgette, and lightweight wool fabrics. It features a classic, unadorned design with a substantial chain and thick quilting without an overt brand logo. Available in light or dark colors of the classic palette: beige, caramel, cognac, brown, ash, graphite, navy, burgundy, or black.

How to Wear

Pair with a cocktail dress for a refined look. Wear with a summer set of trousers and blouse for a chic outfit, or combine with a pleated skirt and silk blouse for added sophistication.

26. Leather Belt

An obligatory complement to pants equipped with loops, this noble addition provides the necessary visual finish to this part of the wardrobe. Made of high-quality natural leather, it is medium-width (corresponding to the size of loops in women's pants) with a subdued classic buckle (devoid of embossing and patterns). It should be well-coordinated in color with the existing wardrobe, adding a refined touch to any outfit.

How to Wear

Pair with pants for a polished look. Wear with a dress to cinch the waist and add definition, or accessorize with a skirt for added elegance.

27. Low-Heeled Court Shoes

In the canon of classic elegance, very high-heeled footwear is not considered particularly chic. Instead, it is replaced with lower models like comfortable pilgrim pump-style court shoes. Adorned with a buckle on a wider, lower heel than a traditional stiletto, and featuring a square toe, these shoes draw on the best traditions of classic footwear. Made of smooth leather for everyday wear or patent leather for more formal occasions.

How to Wear

Pair with a midi skirt and silk blouse for a refined office look. Wear with fabric pants and a turtleneck for a chic outfit, or combine with a dress for added sophistication.

28. Backless Court Shoes

Another stylish type of footwear belonging to the canon of classic elegance, these shoes are an excellent substitute for more formal occasions where sandals and other open-toed models would be too casual. Light in appearance, with a low heel and a strap, they feature an open back but closed toes.

How to Wear

Pair with a cocktail dress for a polished look. Wear with a pleated skirt and blouse for a chic outfit, or combine with trousers and a silk shirt for added elegance.

29. Ballet Flats

A quintessential footwear choice for any elegant Parisienne, ballet flats combine comfort with understated chic. These shoes, typically made from leather or suede, feature a rounded toe and a flat heel, providing style and ease for everyday wear. Available in classic colors such as black, nude, or navy blue, ballet flats are versatile enough to complement any outfit. The minimalistic design often includes a delicate bow on the front, adding a touch of femininity and grace to your steps.

How to Wear

Pair with jeans and a Breton striped t-shirt for a classic French look. Wear with a pleated skirt and blouse for a chic outfit, or combine with a dress for added sophistication.

30. Moccasins

A classic in the casual footwear category, moccasins came from men's wardrobes. Light and unassuming, they are perfect for wearing with trousers like chinos. With a flat sole, covering part of the instep, and featuring buckles or decorative laces, they add much more elegance to outfits than sports shoes like sneakers. In the summer version, often made of lightweight suede, they successfully replace sandals, offering a sophisticated yet relaxed style.

How to Wear

Pair with chinos and a linen shirt for a relaxed look. Wear with fabric pants and a cotton sweater for a casual outfit, or combine with jeans and a turtleneck for added elegance.

31. Chelsea Boots

A footwear classic rooted in men's wardrobes, Chelsea boots are ankle boots with flat heels and slightly rounded toes. They feature characteristic elastic inserts on the sides and decorative stitching and perforations. Although they best complement trousers due to their origin, they can also be paired with wide skirts and midi dresses for a more relaxed yet stylish look.

How to Wear

Pair with jeans and a cotton sweater for a casual look. Wear with a midi skirt and turtleneck for a chic outfit, or combine with fabric pants and a blazer for added sophistication.

32. Classic Ankle Boots

Essential for protection against the cold, classic boots come with a low or slightly higher stable heel and are devoid of unnecessary decorations. They should reach the edge of the garment and cover the calves. If part of the legs is visible under the skirt or dress, thick stockings in the color of the boot upper should be worn.

How to Wear

Pair with a midi skirt and wool coat for a polished winter look. Wear with fabric pants and a turtleneck for a chic outfit, or combine with a dress for added elegance.

33. Elegant Watch

An accessory worth investing in, a chic watch has a timeless shape and unassuming character. Simple, without eccentric decorations, it features a bracelet or leather strap in a classic color that harmonizes with the wardrobe and other accessories. The watch has a round, oval, or rectangular dial, and the case and bracelet color (silver, yellow, or rose gold, two-tone) should match the existing jewelry, adding a touch of sophistication to any outfit.

How to Wear

Pair with a silk blouse and fabric pants for a polished office look. Wear with a dress for added sophistication, or combine with a turtleneck and jeans for a casual yet refined outfit.

34. Classic Ring

A jewel that embodies elegance, the classic ring is essential for an elegant woman. She understands that she does not need many rings. One is enough, especially if it is precious or emotionally significant, inherited from her mother or grandmother. It doesn't need to be extravagant. It can be an engagement ring or a gift to oneself for a milestone birthday, featuring a timeless and classic shape. This ring may showcase a gemstone in white, like a diamond, or in colors like sapphire, ruby, emerald, aquamarine, garnet, citrine, tourmaline, or topaz. Alternatively, it can be adorned with a pearl.

How to Wear

Wear on the ring finger for a subtle touch of elegance. Pair with other minimalist jewelry for a cohesive look, or wear alone as a statement piece.

35. Stylish Earrings

In the jewelry box of an elegant woman, there is always at least one pair of noble earrings. These earrings are classic in shape, not too large, and fastened with English locks, clips, or studs. Made from precious metals in colors that complement the wearer's complexion, eyes, and hair, these earrings might also be adorned with pearls. Whether featuring white or colored gemstones such as diamonds or sapphires, they add elegance, making them suitable for any occasion, from casual outings to formal events.

How to Wear

Pair with a cocktail dress for a refined look. Wear with a blouse and skirt for a chic outfit, or combine with a turtleneck and fabric pants for added sophistication.

French Chic in Everyday Outfits

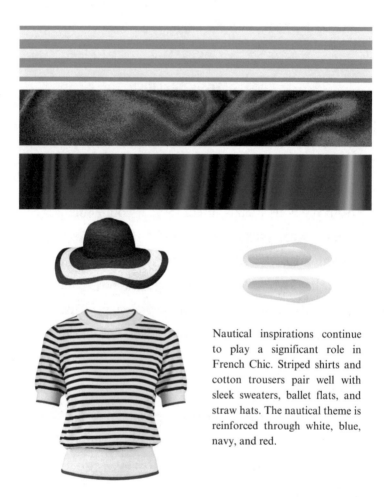

Nautical inspirations continue to play a significant role in French Chic. Striped shirts and cotton trousers pair well with sleek sweaters, ballet flats, and straw hats. The nautical theme is reinforced through white, blue, navy, and red.

French Chic in Everyday Outfits

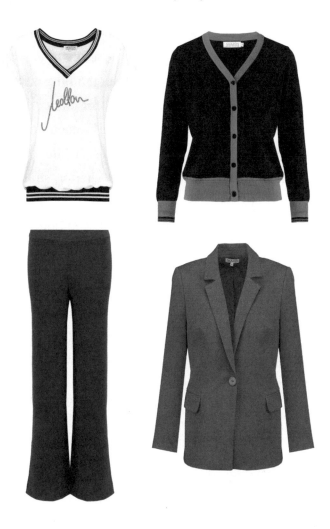

36. Pearl Necklace

A pearl necklace is a timeless addition to an elegant woman's jewelry collection. A short strand of small or medium-sized pearls can brilliantly illuminate the face and add radiance. Pearls, adhering to the canon of classic chic, can be worn from morning onwards. They are recommended not only for mature women but also for young ladies. Mature women might opt for larger and longer necklaces, while younger women are advised to choose shorter strands of smaller beads. The classic white color of pearls ensures a timeless and elegant addition to any ensemble.

How to Wear

Pair with a little black dress for a classic look. Wear with a silk blouse and pleated skirt for a chic outfit, or combine with a turtleneck and jeans for added elegance.

37. Elegant Sunglasses

An essential accessory for adding a touch of glamour and mystery, elegant sunglasses are a must-have in any chic wardrobe. These sunglasses not only protect your eyes from the sun but also serve as a bold fashion statement. Featuring large frames in classic shapes like the cat-eye or round, and available in colors such as black, tortoiseshell, or dark brown, they exude sophistication. The oversized lenses offer maximum coverage, adding elegance to your look whether you're strolling through the city or lounging at a café.

How to Wear

Pair with a trench coat and jeans for a chic daytime look. Wear with a summer dress for added sophistication, or combine with a blouse and skirt for a polished outfit.

38. Vintage Heirloom

Among the cherished possessions of an elegant Parisian woman is a treasured vintage heirloom, inherited from her mother or grandmother. This item, whether a piece of jewelry, a silk scarf, or an ornate brooch, holds a special place in her heart and wardrobe. Rich with history and sentiment, it adds a unique and personal touch to her style. She wears it not just as a fashion statement but as a tribute to her family's legacy and the timeless elegance passed down through generations. This heirloom, carefully preserved and often worn on special occasions, connects her to her roots and enhances her chic, sophisticated look with a touch of nostalgia and tradition.

How to Wear

Pair with a cocktail dress for a refined look. Wear with a blouse and skirt for a chic outfit, or combine with a turtleneck and fabric pants for added sophistication.

39. Red Lipstick

No elegant Parisian woman's beauty arsenal is complete without her favorite red lipstick. This iconic cosmetic item is her secret weapon, instantly elevating her look with glamour. A shade of red that complements her complexion can range from a bold, vibrant crimson to a deep, sophisticated burgundy. Applied with precision, it adds confidence and a classic touch to her appearance, making it perfect for both day and evening looks. This timeless beauty essential is always within reach, whether she's heading to a casual café or an evening event.

How to Wear

Pair with a little black dress for a classic look. Wear with a blouse and skirt for a chic outfit, or combine with a turtleneck and jeans for added elegance.

40. Favorite Perfume

An elegant Parisian woman is known for her signature scent, a perfume she has been faithful to for years. This fragrance is more than just a scent; it is a part of her identity, leaving a subtle but unforgettable impression. Chosen for its timeless and sophisticated notes, it complements her style and personality. Whether a classic French perfume with floral, woody, or musky undertones, it is always applied with a light touch, adding an invisible yet powerful element to her overall elegance.

How to Wear

Apply lightly for a subtle yet memorable touch. Pair with any outfit to add an aura of sophistication and elegance.

French Chic in Everyday Outfits

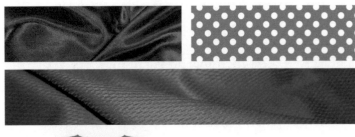

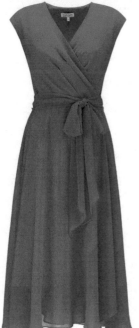

A cocktail dress (here in a sleeveless and red design) can have a more or less formal character, depending on the accessories. Paired with a fitted jacket, it creates a serious image. Combined with a cardigan, it is suitable for more casual occasions. Classic red looks good with black, white, and navy blue.

French Chic in Everyday Outfits

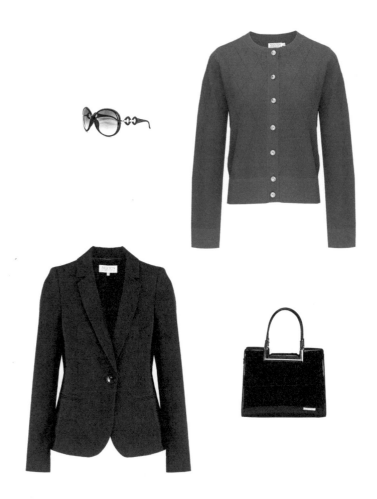

IX.

French Chic Styling Tips
for Different Seasons

French Chic is a timeless style that adapts effortlessly to each season, allowing you to maintain elegance and simplicity year-round. Here are some styling tips for incorporating French Chic into your wardrobe for spring, summer, autumn, and winter. By adapting these tips for each season, you can maintain the effortless elegance that defines French Chic, no matter the weather.

Spring: Fresh and Floral

Key Elements

Lightweight Fabrics: Opt for materials like cotton, linen, and light knits. These fabrics are breathable and perfect for the mild spring weather.

Neutral Palette with Pops of Color: Stick to a base of neutral colors such as white, beige, and soft grey.

French Chic in Everyday Outfits

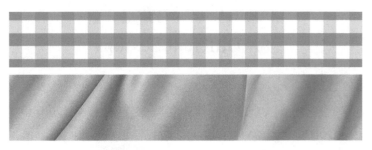

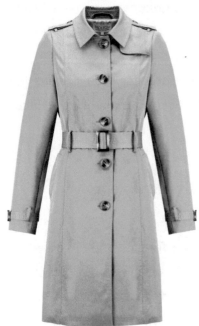

The trench coat, an essential piece for spring and autumn, looks best with trousers. On warmer days, it can be replaced by a blazer. Lime green color pairs interestingly with blue and navy.

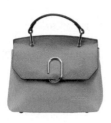

French Chic in Everyday Outfits

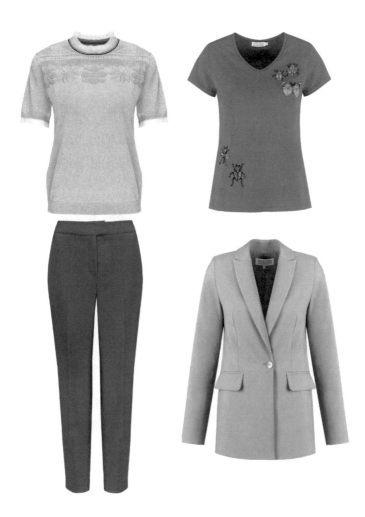

Add subtle pops of pastel colors or delicate floral prints to reflect the season.

Layering: Spring weather can be unpredictable. Layer a light trench coat over a simple blouse and tailored trousers or a midi skirt.

Styling Tips

Trench Coats: A classic beige trench coat is a spring staple. It's versatile and can be paired with almost anything in your wardrobe.

Floral Dresses: Choose a knee-length floral dress and pair it with ballet flats or espadrilles for a chic yet casual look.

Light Scarves: Add a light, silk scarf in a pastel hue to your outfit. It's a simple accessory that can elevate your look instantly.

Cultural Insight

French women often visit local markets for fresh flowers and seasonal produce, reflecting their appreciation for the renewal that spring brings.

Summer: Effortless Elegance

Key Elements

Breathable Fabrics: Stick to natural fabrics like linen, cotton, and lightweight silk to stay cool.

Light and Airy Styles: Opt for relaxed silhouettes such as flowing dresses, wide-leg trousers, and loose tops.

Minimalist Accessories: Keep accessories simple and functional, like a straw hat or a woven basket bag.

Styling Tips

Linen Shirts and Shorts: Pair a white linen shirt with high-waisted shorts. Tuck in the shirt and accessorize with a thin leather belt.

Maxi Dresses: A flowy, neutral-colored maxi dress is perfect for summer. Pair with simple sandals and a delicate necklace.

Espadrilles: Comfortable and stylish, espadrilles are summer footwear essential. They add a touch of French Riviera charm to any outfit.

Summer in France often involves vacations on the coast or strolls through city parks. French women's summer wardrobes reflect a blend of practicality and relaxed elegance suitable for these activities.

Autumn: Cozy and Chic

Key Elements

Transitional Pieces: Use lightweight sweaters, blazers, and trench coats to transition from warmer to cooler weather.

Earthy Tones: Incorporate a palette of earthy tones like camel, olive, burgundy, and navy.

Textured Fabrics: Opt for cozy fabrics such as wool, cashmere, and tweed.

Styling Tips

Blazers: A tailored blazer in a neutral tone can be paired with jeans and a simple tee for a smart casual look.

Scarves and Boots: A wool scarf and ankle boots add warmth and style to any autumn outfit.

Layering: Combine a turtleneck sweater with a midi skirt and finish with a trench coat for a chic layered look.

Cultural Insight

Autumn in Paris is known for its picturesque scenery. Paris often enjoy outdoor cafés and cultural activities, influencing their choice of practical yet stylish attire.

Winter: Warmth and Sophistication

Key Elements

Layering for Warmth: Use multiple layers to stay warm while maintaining a sleek silhouette.

Rich Fabrics: Choose luxurious fabrics such as wool, cashmere, and velvet.

Elegant Outerwear: Invest in a high-quality coat that combines warmth with style.

Styling Tips

Wool Coats: A long, tailored wool coat in a classic color like black, navy, or camel is a winter must-have.

Cashmere Sweaters: Soft cashmere sweaters are both warm and elegant. Pair with tailored trousers or a pencil skirt.

Boots: Knee-high boots or ankle boots are perfect for winter. Choose sleek designs.

Cultural Insight

Winter in Paris often involves visits to museums, holiday markets, and festive gatherings. French women's winter wardrobes are designed to keep them stylish and comfortable in these settings.

X.

The Colors of French Chic

The essence of French chic lies in its ability to blend simplicity with elegance, and colors play a crucial role in this balance. French women tend to favor neutral and classic colors, using bold hues sparingly to enhance their outfits. The careful selection and combination of colors reflect a deep understanding of style and an appreciation for timeless fashion.

The colors of the French flag – blue, white, and red – hold deep symbolic significance and have left an indelible mark on French fashion and the concept of "French chic." Blue represents liberty, white symbolizes equality, and red signifies fraternity. These values are mirrored in the elegance and sophistication of French fashion, where colors play a crucial role in defining style and personality.

Blue: The Color of Liberty

Blue, a color often associated with depth and stability, is a staple in the wardrobes of many Parisians. Navy blue, in particular, is a favorite. It exudes calm sophistication and pairs effortlessly with almost any other color. French women often incorporate navy blue into their wardrobes through classic pieces like trench coats, blazers, and sweaters. It's a versatile hue transition seamlessly from day to night, making it a cornerstone of French chic.

White: The Symbol of Elegance and Purity

White is synonymous with elegance and purity in French fashion. It's a color that stands out for its simplicity and timelessness. French women love white blouses, crisp white shirts, and tailored white trousers. In the summer, white linen dresses and skirts are popular choices, offering a fresh and clean look. White in an outfit can create a striking contrast when paired with darker colors, highlighting the simplicity and elegance integral to French chic.

Red: The Color of Passion and Confidence

Red is the color of passion, confidence, and boldness. It's often used as an accent color to add a touch of drama and vibrancy to an outfit. French women might choose a red dress for a special occasion or add a pop of red with accessories like scarves, handbags, or shoes. A red lipstick is also a classic choice that adds a sophisticated flair to any look, embodying the confident spirit of French women.

Elegant Color Combinations Favored by Parisians

Parisians are masters of mixing and matching colors to create effortlessly chic looks. Here are some elegant color combinations that are particularly favored:

Navy Blue and White

This combination is a timeless classic. It's fresh, clean, and sophisticated. A navy blazer paired with white trousers or a navy striped shirt with white jeans is quintessentially French.

The Colors of French Chic

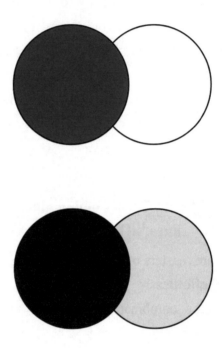

Elegant color combinations that are particularly favored by Parisians: navy blue and white, black and beige, grey and camel, red and navy blue, burgundy and blush pink.

The Colors of French Chic

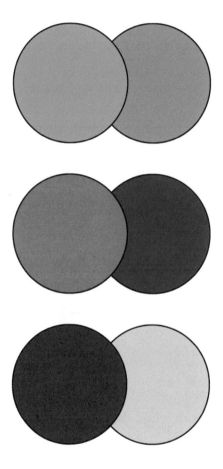

Black and Beige

Black is a dominant color in French fashion due to its versatility and slimming effect. Paired with beige, it creates a chic, understated look. A black dress with a beige coat is a perfect example of this combination.

Grey and Camel

These neutral tones complement each other beautifully. A grey sweater paired with camel trousers or a camel coat over a grey dress is a sophisticated and stylish choice.

Red and Navy Blue

For a bolder look, red and navy make a striking combination. A red scarf or handbag paired with a navy outfit adds a touch of vibrancy without being overwhelming.

Burgundy and Blush Pink

This is a more modern and romantic combination. Burgundy, a rich and deep color, pairs wonderfully with the softness of blush pink. It's perfect for autumn and winter, creating a warm and elegant look.

XI.

Makeup and Hairstyles
in French Chic Style

The French Chic style is synonymous with elegance, simplicity, and naturalness. This approach to fashion and beauty emphasizes the individual beauty of each woman without overdoing it. The key to achieving this look is natural makeup and hairstyles that appear effortless, though they are meticulously planned and executed.

The essence of French chic makeup and hairstyles lies in the balance between effortlessness and sophistication. French women master the art of looking polished without appearing overdone, embracing their natural beauty with subtle enhancements.

This timeless approach to beauty makes the French chic style so universally admired and emulated.

Makeup in French Chic Style

Natural Base

French women prioritize a healthy and radiant complexion. Instead of a heavy foundation, they opt for light, breathable products that even out the skin tone without masking its natural texture. BB creams or light-coverage foundations are popular choices, paired with a touch of concealer to cover any imperfections.

Subtle Eyes

The eyes are often understated yet defined. A light sweep of neutral eyeshadow enhances the natural contours of the eyes. Eyeliner is used sparingly, typically in a soft brown or charcoal shade, to accentuate the lash line. Mascara is essential, applied in one or two coats to lengthen and define the lashes without clumping.

Rosy Cheeks

Blush is crucial for that fresh, healthy glow. French women prefer cream or liquid blushes that blend seamlessly into the skin, giving a natural flush. Shades of peach, rose, and soft pink are the go-to colors, applied lightly to the apples of the cheeks.

Classic Lips

Lip color is where French women often make a statement. The classic red lip is iconic, but it also embraces softer shades like nude, rose, and coral for a more subdued look. The key is to keep the lips hydrated and defined, often opting for a satin or matte finish.

Hairstyles in French Chic Style

Effortless Waves

The quintessential French hairstyle is the "effortless waves." This look is achieved by using minimal styling products and tools, focusing on enhancing the hair's natural texture. A bit of sea salt spray can add volume and texture, creating soft, tousled waves that look chic and carefree.

Elegant Buns and Chignons

For more formal occasions, French women often choose elegant updos like low buns or chignons. These hairstyles are typically loose and slightly undone, avoiding the overly polished look. A few strands left free around the face add a touch of softness and romance.

Natural Straight Hair

Straight hair, when styled the French way, is never pin-straight. It's usually left with a bit of natural wave or texture. French women embrace their hair's natural state, enhancing it with light styling to keep it looking fresh and effortless.

Bangs (Fringe)

Bangs are a staple in French hairstyles. Whether blunt, wispy, or curtain-style, bangs add an element of sophistication and youthfulness. They are usually styled to look natural, with a slight wave or texture.

Minimalist Approach

The overarching theme in French chic hairstyles is minimalism. French women avoid heavy styling products and elaborate techniques. Instead, they focus on keeping their hair healthy and well-maintained, letting its natural beauty shine through.

XII.

French Chic and Personal Identity

French Chic transcends mere fashion trends. It is a celebration of individuality and personal expression. Rooted in simplicity, elegance, and a keen sense of self, French Chic encourages women to embrace their unique identities while adhering to timeless fashion principles.

By embracing these principles of French Chic, you can develop a personal style that is both elegant and uniquely yours. It is about finding the balance between timeless fashion and personal expression, creating a wardrobe that reflects your identity and makes you feel confident every day.

Embracing Authenticity

Key Elements

Self-Discovery: Understanding your personal preferences, body shape, and lifestyle is the first step toward developing a unique style. French women are renowned for their deep self-awareness, which guides their fashion choices.

Simplicity and Subtlety: French Chic emphasizes understated elegance. Opting for simple, well-tailored garments allows your personality to stand out without being eclipsed by your attire.

Styling Tips

Signature Pieces: Identify crucial pieces that reflect your personality. Whether it is a classic trench coat, a perfectly tailored blazer, or a beloved pair of jeans, make these items the cornerstone of your wardrobe.

Personal Touches: Incorporate accessories that have personal significance, such as vintage jewelry, a scarf from a memorable trip, or a handbag that holds sentimental value.

Cultural Insight

French women often inherit fashion sensibilities from their mothers or grandmothers, incorporating vintage pieces into their modern wardrobes. This blending of old and new creates a deeply personal and unique style.

Curating a Thoughtful Wardrobe

Key Elements

Quality over Quantity: Invest in high-quality, timeless pieces that will last. French Chic is about having fewer, better items that you love and wear frequently.

Versatility: Choose items that can be mixed and matched easily. A garderobe of a French woman is typically versatile, allowing for outfits from a limited number of pieces.

Styling Tips

Capsule Wardrobe: Create a capsule wardrobe consisting of essential items that reflect your style. It might include a white blouse, black trousers, a little black dress, a neutral blazer, and classic jeans.

Seasonal Updates: Refresh your wardrobe each season by adding new pieces that fit with your existing items. It keeps your style current without losing its core identity.

Cultural Insight

French women are known for their discerning eye for detail. They often frequent small boutiques and local markets, where they find unique, high-quality pieces that add character to their wardrobes.

Expressing Individuality through Fashion

Key Elements

Personal Style: While French Chic has its rules, it also celebrates breaking them in favor of expression. Do not be afraid to experiment and find what makes you feel most confident.

Confidence: True French Chic is less about the clothes themselves and more about the attitude with which they are worn. Confidence is the basis for pulling off any look.

Styling Tips

Experimentation: Try different combinations and style to see what resonates with you. Do not be afraid to step out of your comfort zone occasionally.

Signature Look: Develop a signature look that people associate with you. It could be a specific color palette, a favorite accessory, or a silhouette that flatters your figure.

Iconic French women like Coco Chanel, Brigitte Bardot, and Jane Birkin are celebrated for their distinct personal styles. Each took elements of French Chic and made them their own, inspiring generations of women to do the same.

The Role of Accessories

Key Elements

Minimalism with Impact: Accessories in French Elegance are used sparingly but purposefully. They should complement the outfit without overwhelming it.

Meaningful Choices: Opt for accessories that have personal meaning or add a unique touch to your outfit.

Styling Tips

Scarves and Hats: A silk scarf or a chic beret can add a French touch to any outfit. Experiment with different ways to tie a scarf or styles of hats that suit your face shape.

Jewelry: Choose delicate, understated jewelry. A pair of pearl earrings, a simple gold bracelet, or a classic watch can add a touch of elegance to your look.

Cultural Insight

French women often favor heirloom jewelry or pieces that tell a story, adding a layer of personal history and meaning to their style.

Fashion as a Form of Self-Care

Key Elements

Mindful Dressing: Taking the time to dress well is seen as a form of self-respect and self-care. It is about feeling good in what you wear and presenting yourself with confidence.

Comfort and Style: French Chic does not sacrifice comfort for style. Finding pieces that feel as good as they look is crucial.

Styling Tips

Daily Rituals: Incorporate a daily dressing ritual that makes you feel good. It could be as simple as choosing your outfit the night before or taking a few extra minutes to accessorize.

Comfortable Elegance: Look for stylish pieces that are also comfortable, like well-fitted jeans with a touch of stretch or a soft cashmere sweater.

Cultural Insight

The concept of *bien dans sa peau* (feeling good in one's skin) is central to French culture. It is about enhancing your natural beauty through fashion and lifestyle choices.

By embracing these principles of French Chic, you can develop a personal style that is both elegant and uniquely yours. It is about finding the balance between timeless fashion and personal expression, creating a wardrobe that reflects your identity and makes you feel confident every day.

XIII.

How Women in Paris
Dress for Different Events

Parisian women are renowned for their ability to tailor their outfits to various occasions. Whether they're heading to a casual meeting, a grand event, dinner, a date, or a business meeting, they always present themselves impeccably. Their secret lies in simplicity, elegance, and a keen sense of style, allowing them to look always appropriate and chic. Inspired by their style, we can learn how to create sophisticated outfits from simple elements for any occasion.

Everyday Meetings

Everyday life in Paris is a constant balance between comfort and elegance. Parisian women have mastered the art of combining these two qualities, creating outfits that are not only practical but also stylish. For everyday meetings, such as coffee with a friend, shopping, or a walk in the park, they choose clothes that allow them to feel comfortable while still looking fashionable.

Everyday Outfits

Basic Wardrobe Elements

- Jeans: High-quality jeans in classic cuts, such as slim fit or straight leg, are the cornerstone of a Parisian woman's daily wardrobe. They often choose darker shades that are easy to pair with various tops.

- T-shirts and Blouses: Simple white T-shirts are essential. Parisian women also appreciate silk blouses in neutral colors, which add elegance to their outfits.

- Sweaters: A light cashmere sweater or cardigan is the perfect addition for cooler days. They often choose classic shades like beige, navy, or gray.

Layers and Outerwear

- Blazers: A well-tailored blazer is a must-have. Parisian women often wear them even with casual outfits to add a touch of elegance.

- Trench Coats: A classic beige trench coat is an icon of French fashion. It's perfect for spring and autumn, adding a hint of Parisian chic to any outfit.

- Coats: In winter, they opt for wool coats in neutral colors that are warm and stylish.

Footwear

- Ballet Flats: Classic ballet flats are comfortable and match most everyday outfits. Black, beige, or subtly patterned, they are an indispensable part of the wardrobe.

- Ankle Boots: Leather ankle boots with a low heel are ideal for colder days. Parisian women choose models that are both comfortable and elegant.

- Sneakers: In recent years, Parisian women have opted increasingly for stylish sneakers, which they pair with more elegant wardrobe elements to create beautiful contrasts.

Accessories

- Bags: A leather bag is fundamental. Parisian women often choose classic models, such as shoulder bags or small, elegant crossbody bags.

- Jewelry: Minimalist jewelry, like delicate gold earrings, subtle bracelets, or an elegant watch, adds class and sophistication to an outfit.

- Sunglasses: Stylish sunglasses, often in a vintage style, are an essential element of daily outfits, adding a touch of mystery and glamour.

Details

- Scarves and Shawls: A light silk scarf or cotton shawl can transform any outfit. Parisian women often choose subtle patterns and colors that match the rest of their wardrobe.

- Hats and Caps: On cooler days, they opt for stylish berets, and for spring and summer – straw hats that add character and protect from the sun.

Sample Everyday Outfits

For a Walk in the Park

- Outfit: Simple jeans, white T-shirt, light cashmere sweater, trench coat, ballet flats.

- Accessories: Small leather shoulder bag, gold earrings, sunglasses.

For Coffee with a Friend

- Outfit: Slim fit jeans, silk blouse in a neutral color, blazer, sneakers.

- Accessories: Minimalist jewelry, elegant watch, silk scarf.

For Shopping

- Outfit: Straight-leg jeans, plain T-shirt, cardigan, leather ankle boots.

- Accessories: Stylish crossbody bag, beret, light shawl.

Romantic Meetings

Dates in Paris are special moments, full of magic and romance. Parisian women know how to highlight their beauty and personality to enchant their partner. Whether it's a first meeting or dinner with a long-time partner, Parisian women pay attention to every detail of their outfits, creating a look that is both seductive and elegant.

Date Outfits

First Date

- Dresses: For a first date, Parisian women often choose dresses that highlight their natural charm but are not overly provocative. These can be romantic floral dresses or little black dresses.

- Materials: Cotton, silk, and linen – natural materials that are comfortable and look elegant.

- Shoes: Comfortable yet stylish shoes, such as ballet flats or low-heeled pumps.

- Accessories: Delicate jewelry, such as a subtle necklace and earrings, and a small shoulder bag.

Restaurant Date

- Outfit: For an elegant dinner at a restaurant, Parisian women may choose more sophisticated attire. It could be silk dresses or stylish suits.

- Dresses: Cocktail dresses, often in classic colors like black, navy, or red, highlight elegance and sensuality.

- Shoes: Heels or elegant heeled sandals that add grace and charm.

- Accessories: High-quality jewelry, such as pearls or gold earrings, and an elegant clutch.

Outdoor Date

- Outfit: For outdoor dates, like a walk in the park or a picnic, Parisian women choose outfits that combine comfort with romance.

- Clothes: Flowy dresses in pastel colors, stylish jeans, and blouses with lace details.

- Shoes: Comfortable shoes, such as ballet flats, espadrilles, or stylish sneakers.

- Accessories: Straw hat, large sunglasses, delicate jewelry, and a practical yet elegant bag.

Sample Date Outfits

First Date

- Outfit: Romantic floral dress, beige ballet flats, subtle necklace, and small shoulder bag.

- Accessories: Delicate earrings, natural makeup, light scarf.

Restaurant Date

- Outfit: Navy blue silk cocktail dress, black heels, pearl earrings, and elegant clutch.

- Accessories: Gold bracelet, red lips, subtle perfume.

Outdoor Date

- Outfit: Flowy pastel dress, espadrilles, straw hat, large sunglasses.

- Accessories: Small crossbody bag, delicate bracelet, light makeup.

French Chic in Everyday Outfits

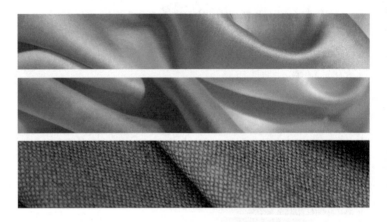

A woman's suit creates a trustworthy image. To soften the look, you can wear its pieces separately. Suit trousers look great with a plain blazer and a silk blouse. Burgundy looks very noble with blush pink, beige, and brown.

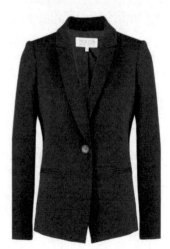

French Chic in Everyday Outfits

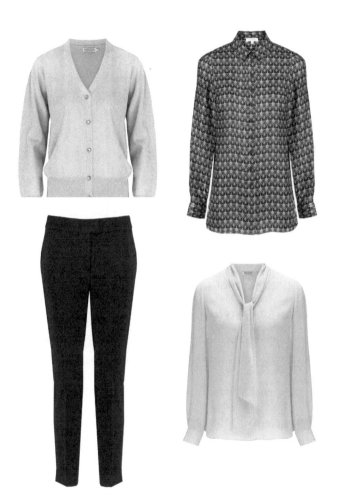

Business Meetings

Professional meetings allow Parisian women to showcase their professionalism and elegance. They understand the importance of first impressions, so they pay attention to every detail of their appearance. They choose outfits that combine classic elegance with modern, business chic. Here is how they prepare for such events.

Elements of Business Attire

Suits and Jumpsuits

- Suits: Classic, well-tailored suits are essential. Parisian women choose traditional colors like navy, black, or gray and bolder ones like burgundy or bottle green.

- Jumpsuits: Stylish jumpsuits are an alternative to the classic suit. Made from elegant fabrics, they work perfectly for formal meetings.

Dresses and Skirts

- Dresses: Simple, classic pencil dresses in muted colors are a safe choice. They must be well-fitted and made from high-quality materials.

- Skirts: Pencil skirts paired with elegant blouses are a classic set. Parisian women often choose

144

models with light patterns or textures that add character to the outfit.

Blouses and Shirts

- Blouses: Silk blouses in neutral colors or delicate patterns are elegant and feminine. Parisian women often choose models with subtle details, such as bows or delicate embroidery.

- Shirts: Classic white shirts are a must-have. They can be paired with suits and skirts, creating a professional look.

Shoes

- Pumps: Classic pumps with a small heel are comfortable and elegant. Parisian women often choose models in black, nude, or navy.

- Ballet Flats: For less formal meetings, stylish ballet flats are a perfect choice.

Accessories

- Bags: Elegant leather bags in classic colors. Parisian women choose models that are both stylish and practical.

- Jewelry: Subtle jewelry, such as delicate earrings, minimalist bracelets, or elegant watches. They avoid excessive accessories, opting for chic simplicity.

- Belts: Thin leather belts can add character to a suit or dress, accentuating the waist.

Sample Business Meeting Outfits

Suit

- Outfit: Navy blue suit, white silk blouse, black pumps, leather bag in nude color.
- Accessories: Silver earrings, minimalist watch, delicate necklace.

Dress

- Outfit: Black pencil dress, beige jacket, black ballet flats, elegant bag.
- Accessories: Gold earrings, subtle bracelet, leather belt at the waist.

Jumpsuit

- Outfit: Bottle green jumpsuit, black pumps, small leather shoulder bag.
- Accessories: Pearl earrings, delicate ring, elegant belt.

Hairstyle and Makeup

- Hairstyle: Parisian women opt for elegant but natural hairstyles. It can be straight, smooth hair, delicate waves, or elegant updos. The hairstyle must be neat and professional.

- Makeup: Natural yet sophisticated. The skin should look fresh and radiant, with a subtle emphasis on the eyes and lips. Red lips, though classic, are less often chosen for business meetings – Parisian women prefer neutral shades.

Grand Event

Special occasions are a perfect opportunity to showcase the best fashion creations. Parisian women, known for their elegance and refined style, excel at preparing for special occasions, such as galas, film premieres, operas, or exclusive banquets. Here is how they prepare.

Elements of Grand Event Outfits

Evening Dresses

- Long Dresses: Parisian women often choose long, elegant dresses in classic colors like black, navy, or red. These can be dresses with subtle embellishments, such as lace, sequins, or delicate embroidery.

- Cocktail Dresses: For less formal events, they opt for stylish cocktail dresses, often with chic cuts or details.

Materials and Details

- Materials: High-quality fabrics are key. Silk, satin, velvet, and lace are frequent choices.
- Details: Parisian women love delicate elements, such as elegant necklines, bare backs, or chic slits. They avoid excessive embellishments, preferring subtle elegance.

Shoes

- Heels: High heels are essential for grand events. Parisian women choose elegant pumps or sandals that match the dress.
- Comfort: Despite the height of the heel, comfort is crucial. Shoes should be well-fitted and allow for comfortable movement.

Accessories

- Jewelry: High-quality jewelry is a must-have. Parisian women choose chic earrings, necklaces, or bracelets that complement their outfits. They often opt for diamonds, pearls, or gold jewelry.

- Bags: A small clutch is the perfect choice. It should be elegant and match the overall look.

- Shawls and Stoles: For cooler evenings, Parisian women often choose stylish shawls or stoles made from high-quality materials, such as silk.

Sample Grand Event Outfits

Opera Gala

- Outfit: Long, navy blue satin dress with a bare back, black high-heeled sandals, small clutch.

- Accessories: Diamond earrings, delicate bracelet, cashmere shawl.

Film Premiere

- Outfit: Stylish red cocktail dress with a deep neckline, black pumps, small gold clutch.

- Accessories: Pearl necklace, gold bracelet.

Exclusive Banquet

- Outfit: Black velvet long dress with lace details, nude high-heeled sandals, small black clutch.

- Accessories: Silver earrings, diamond ring, silk stole.

French Chic in Everyday Outfits

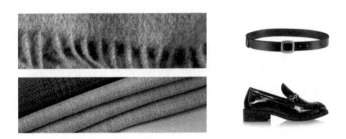

A smoothly woven sweater in a classic cut is versatile, much like a sleek turtleneck. Both wardrobe pieces pair well with dark jeans or tailored trousers. Completing such an outfit are a leather belt, flat shoes, and a short woolen coat. Ash gray looks beautiful with black, white, and navy blue.

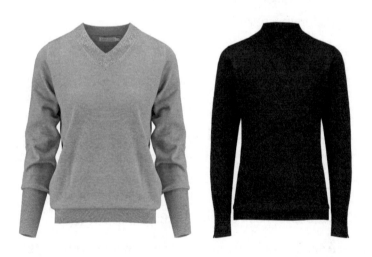

French Chic in Everyday Outfits

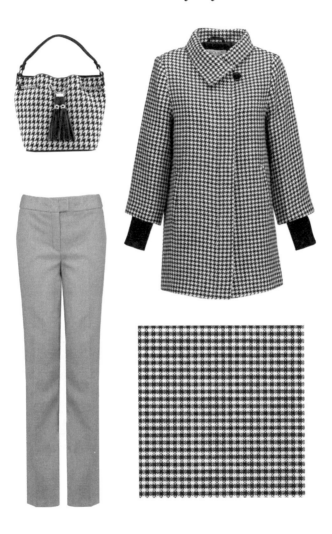

XIV.

Parisian Ladies on Style and French Chic

In the vibrant streets of Paris, amidst its timeless architecture and bustling cafés, Parisian women effortlessly embody a style that has captivated the world for generations. Their approach to fashion transcends fleeting trends. It is a way of life steeped in elegance, individuality, and an appreciation for craftsmanship.

Each woman brings a unique interpretation of French chic, a reflection of her profession, personal preferences, and timeless style sensibilities. Join us as we explore the perspectives of these ten Parisian women who graciously shared their insights on style and the essence of French chic. Let's delve into their stories and uncover the allure of Parisian elegance through their eyes.

Chantal, 43, Architect

"For me, French chic is about simplicity and elegance. As an architect, my work demands creativity and precision, and I like my outfits to reflect the same. I often opt for classic blazers and tailored trousers, which offer both style and comfort. My go-to piece is a silk button-up blouse, which adds a touch of sophistication without being over the top. I believe that the right accessories, like a timeless watch and a statement ring, can elevate any look. French chic is about feeling confident and polished, whether I'm meeting clients or working on-site."

Favorite Wardrobe Item: Classic blazer

Cannot Do Without: Silk button-up blouse

Favorite Color: White

Favorite Designer or French Brand: Yves Saint Laurent

Advice for Women Wanting to Achieve French Chic: Invest in well-tailored classics and remember to accessorize elegantly.

Sophie, 36, Publishing House Employee

"French chic is all about understated elegance and being true to yourself. In my job at the publishing house, I need to look professional but also creative. I love wearing a pleated skirt with a smooth turtleneck or a classic cardigan. These pieces are versatile and can be dressed up or down depending on the occasion. For me, a pair of low-heeled court shoes and a classic handbag are essential. They provide comfort and style, allowing me to move seamlessly from a meeting to a casual lunch with authors. French chic is about blending comfort with elegance in a way that feels uniquely me."

Favorite Wardrobe Item: Pleated skirt

Cannot Do Without: Classic handbag

Favorite Color: Navy blue

Favorite Designer or French Brand: Chloé

Advice for Women Wanting to Achieve French Chic: Focus on quality over quantity. Choose versatile pieces that are easy to mix and match.

French Chic in Everyday Outfits

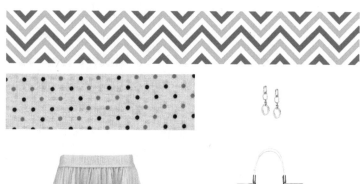

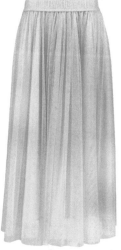

The pleated skirt is a classic wardrobe staple favored by Parisians. Spring and summer styles are light, making them perfect to combine with lightweight pieces such as blouses, thin sweaters, and light blazers. Blush pink looks great not only with burgundy but also with white, ecru, and green.

French Chic in Everyday Outfits

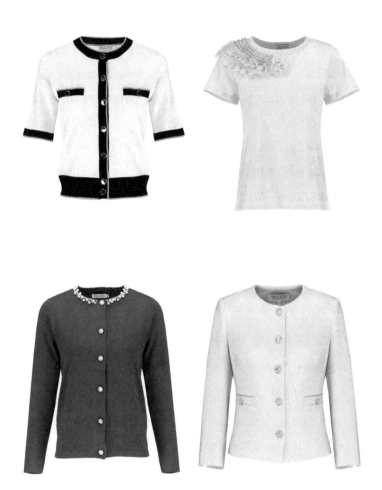

Mila, 29, Content Manager
in an Advertising Agency

"Working in advertising means I need to balance professionalism with creativity. French chic helps me achieve that balance. I often wear a classic blazer with dark jeans or chinos, which looks stylish and is perfect for the dynamic nature of my job. I love adding a pop of color with a bold accessory or red lipstick. My style is all about mixing modern pieces with timeless classics. French chic allows me to express my individuality while maintaining a polished and professional appearance."

Favorite Wardrobe Item: Classic blazer

Cannot Do Without: Red lipstick

Favorite Color: Black

Favorite Designer or French Brand: Isabel Marant

Advice for Women Wanting to Achieve French Chic: Don't be afraid to add a splash of color to classic outfits. It adds character and individuality.

Chloé, 48, Secretary in a Law Firm

"In my role at the law firm, French chic is about maintaining a professional and composed image. I prefer classic and well-tailored pieces, like a midi skirt paired with a silk button-up blouse or a wool coat during the colder months. These items are not only stylish but also exude confidence and reliability. I believe that small details, such as a pair of pearl earrings or a vintage brooch, can make a big difference. For me, French chic is about subtle elegance and making a statement through simplicity and quality."

Favorite Wardrobe Item: Wool coat

Cannot Do Without: Pearl earrings

Favorite Color: Grey

Favorite Designer or French Brand: Hermès

Advice for Women Wanting to Achieve French Chic: Pay attention to details and accessories. They often define the entire outfit.

Emma, 69, Homemaker

"Even though I'm retired, French chic still plays a significant role in my daily life. It represents timeless elegance and the joy of looking put-together, no matter the occasion. I enjoy wearing a smooth cardigan with a pair of classic trousers or a cotton sweater with a linen shirt underneath. Comfort is key for me, but I never compromise on style. I cherish my vintage heirlooms like a beautiful silk scarf passed down from my mother, which adds a personal touch to my outfits. French chic is about celebrating femininity and grace at any age."

Favorite Wardrobe Item: Silk scarf

Cannot Do Without: Wool sweater

Favorite Color: Beige

Favorite Designer or French Brand: Dior

Advice for Women Wanting to Achieve French Chic: Invest in timeless accessories that you can wear for many years.

Coralie, 52, Ophthalmologist

"As a doctor, my work attire needs to be practical yet professional. French chic helps me achieve this balance effortlessly. I prefer wearing tailored pieces, like a classic blazer over a smooth turtleneck or a midi skirt. These items are comfortable and professional, allowing me to move easily between consultations. I also love incorporating elegant accessories, such as a stylish watch or a simple ring. French chic, for me, is about looking polished and approachable, reflecting both my professional and personal style."

Favorite Wardrobe Item: Fitted blazer

Cannot Do Without: Stylish watch

Favorite Color: Navy blue

Favorite Designer or French Brand: Givenchy

Advice for Women Wanting to Achieve French Chic: Ensure your clothes are always well-tailored and neat. This is key to an elegant look.

French Chic in Everyday Outfits

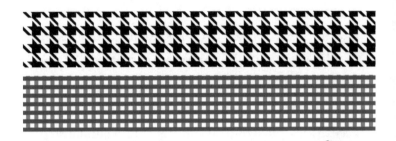

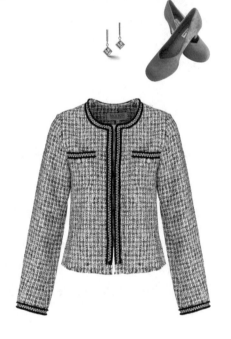

Each component of a classic skirt suit can be worn independently, making the ensemble more casual. The jacket pairs well with plain trousers. The skirt complements a lightweight blazer. The combination of black and white looks beautiful with various shades of blue and gray.

French Chic in Everyday Outfits

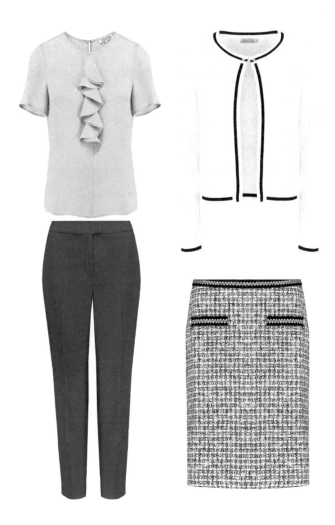

Marie-Louise, 73, Retired Office Worker

"To me, French chic is about embracing timeless elegance and comfort. In my retirement, I prioritize outfits that are both stylish and easy to wear. I love my collection of classic wool coats and elegant silk scarves, which I pair with simple, well-cut trousers and cozy sweaters. These pieces allow me to stay warm and look sophisticated whether I'm out for a walk or meeting friends for coffee. French chic, for me, is about maintaining a refined appearance that feels effortless and true to my style."

Favorite Wardrobe Item: Classic wool coat

Cannot Do Without: Silk scarf

Favorite Color: Burgundy

Favorite Designer or French Brand: Lanvin

Advice for Women Wanting to Achieve French Chic: Stick to classics that are always in style and emphasize your individuality.

Léa, 22, Foreign Languages Student

"French chic is the perfect way to express my personality through fashion. As a student, I often mix casual and classic pieces to create a look that is both stylish and practical for my busy schedule. I love wearing dark jeans with a smooth turtleneck and adding a pop of color with a bright scarf or bold lipstick. My favorite accessories are my vintage jewelry pieces, which I inherited from my grandmother. They add a unique touch to my outfits and make me feel connected to my heritage. French chic is about blending the old with the new in a way that feels fresh and modern."

Favorite Wardrobe Item: Dark jeans

Cannot Do Without: Vintage jewelry

Favorite Color: Red

Favorite Designer or French Brand: A.P.C.

Advice for Women Wanting to Achieve French Chic: Don't hesitate to mix modern elements with classics to create a unique style.

Adrienne, 44, Hotel Receptionist

"In my role at the hotel, French chic is essential for presenting a professional and welcoming image to our guests. I prefer wearing tailored dresses and classic blazers, which give me a polished look while being comfortable enough to wear all day. My go-to pieces include a little black dress for special occasions and a well-fitted blazer for daily wear. I also love accessorizing with simple, elegant jewelry and a classic handbag. French chic is about making a lasting impression with a refined and understated style."

Favorite Wardrobe Item: Little black dress

Cannot Do Without: Classic handbag

Favorite Color: Black

Favorite Designer or French Brand: Balenciaga

Advice for Women Wanting to Achieve French Chic: Classic wardrobe pieces never go out of style. Invest in well-tailored clothes that always look elegant.

Isabelle, 56, Sales Associate in a Cosmetic Store

"Working in the beauty industry, French chic helps me present a polished and stylish appearance to our customers. I often wear classic, monochrome outfits like a silk button-up blouse with a pleated skirt or tailored trousers. These pieces are versatile and allow me to mix and match different elements of my wardrobe. I also enjoy wearing red lipstick and a pair of stylish earrings to add a touch of glamour. For me, French chic is about feeling confident and looking effortlessly put-together, whether I'm at work or enjoying my free time."

Favorite Wardrobe Item: Silk blouse

Cannot Do Without: Red lipstick

Favorite Color: Beige

Favorite Designer or French Brand: Lancôme

Advice for Women Wanting to Achieve French Chic: Remember simplicity and elegance. Sometimes less is more, and attention to detail is crucial.

XV.

Famous Quotes on French Women and Elegance

French women have been made beautiful by the French people – they're very aware of their bodies, the way they move and speak, and they're very confident of their sexuality. French society has made them like that.

Charlotte Rampling,

an English actress and model

French women don't have too many clothes – a few good pieces that last for a while and are classic and timeless.

Mireille Guiliano,

a French-American author

You need mystery. You do. I think that's what foreign women, French women, in particular, are good at.

There's still a sense that you need to keep
some of the unknown because that's where
the soul resides, or something.

Jason Clarke,

an Australian actor

A French woman is a perfect architect in dress:
she never, with Gothic ignorance, mixes the orders;
she never tricks out a snobby Doric shape with
Corinthian finery; or, to speak without metaphor,
she conforms to general fashion only when it
happens not to be repugnant to private beauty.

Oliver Goldsmith,

an Anglo-Irish novelist, dramatist and poet

It's funny because I think that both France and
Britain are known for their distinctive styles and
everyone says that France is so chic and elegant but
I think more than that French women are renowned
for dressing in what suits them.

Alexa Chung,

an English model and television personality

American women often fall into the trap of, "Oh, these are my weekend clothes. These are my work clothes. This is what I wear at night." It's so old-fashioned. The French are not afraid of their luxury. Americans can be so puritanical and think, "That's my special-occasion bag." Whereas, for a French woman, it's her everyday bag.

Michael Kors,

an American fashion designer

Living in Paris was a crash course in chic.

Rebecca Romijn,

an American actress and model

XVI.

20 Tips for Cultivating
French Chic Daily

French Chic is not just a way of dressing but also an approach to life that combines elegance, simplicity, and naturalness. Implementing these practical tips will help you cultivate this timeless aesthetic daily.

1. **Invest in Basics**: Buy high-quality wardrobe staples like well-fitted jeans, a white shirt, and a classic little black dress. These items are timeless and versatile.

2. **Choose Natural Fabrics**: Prefer fabrics such as cotton, wool, silk, and linen, which not only look elegant but are also more durable and comfortable.

3. **Embrace Minimalism**: Avoid excessive styling in clothes and makeup. French Chic is all about

simplicity and elegance without overdoing it.

4. **Perfect Fit is Key**: Ensure your clothes fit perfectly. Consider investing in a tailor to customize your clothes to your measurements.

5. **Always Be Prepared**: Keep a few accessories on hand, like a silk scarf, a classic handbag, and delicate jewelry, which can quickly elevate and transform any outfit.

6. **Skincare First**: Beautiful, healthy skin is the foundation of a natural look. Regularly cleanse, moisturize, and protect your skin from the sun.

7. **Natural Makeup**: Opt for subtle makeup. Light foundation, a touch of mascara, a bit of blush, and the iconic red lipstick are the essence of French Chic.

8. **Effortless Hairstyle**: Care for your hair, but avoid over-styling. Lightly tousled natural waves or a simple chignon add elegance

without looking artificial.

9. **Highlight One Element**: In outfit, emphasize one standout element, such as a unique necklace, a colorful scarf, or a designer bag.

10. **Comfort and Style**: Your clothes should be both stylish and comfortable. French Chic is primarily about combining comfort with elegance.

11. **Attention to Details**: Carefully chosen buttons, precise seams, and well-matched accessories can make the simplest outfit look exceptional.

12. **Classic Colors**: Use neutral colors like black, white, gray, and beige. They are easy to mix and always look elegant.

13. **Avoid Logos**: Subtlety is key to French Chic. Avoid clothing and accessories with large, flashy logos.

14. **Pay Attention to Footwear**: Good quality shoes are the foundation of any outfit. Choose classic models that are both stylish and comfortable.

15. **Find Your Style**: French Chic is about authenticity. Find fashion elements that best express your personality and stick with them.

16. **Care for Your Clothes**: Remember to properly care for your clothes. Regular washing, ironing, and storage will keep them looking new for a long time.

17. **Minimalist Jewelry**: Opt for minimalist, delicate jewelry. Often, a single well-chosen bracelet or pair of earrings is enough to add elegance.

18. **Perfume as an Accent**: Use subtle, classic perfumes. The scent should complement your personality, not dominate it.

19. **Inspiration from Nature**: Draw inspiration from nature. Earth tones, botanical motifs, and natural materials always fit into the French Chic style.

20. **Confidence**: The most important element of French Chic is confidence. Wearing your clothes with pride and ease will always make you look stylish and elegant.

List of Illustrations

p. 16-17: Dresses from the Musée Galliera, Wikimedia.org.

p. 18-19: Images from Unsplash.com, Pixabay.com. Chanel's portrait: Wikimedia.org. Photo bottom right on page 18: dress from Rhode Island School of Design Museum of Art, Wikimedia.org.

p. 20-21: Images from Unsplash.com. Photo bottom left on page 20: Wikimedia.org.

p. 24-25: Photos from the Dutch National Archives, Wikimedia.org.

p. 30, 31, 36, 37: Images from Unsplash.com, Pixabay.com.

p. 50-51: Photos from Wikimedia.org.

p. 58-59: Images on the top on page 58: Unsplash.com. Photos with the models: Bialcon, press materials, Tweed.pl.

p. 74-75: Skirt: Bialcon, press materials, Tweed.pl. Other clothing packshots: Molton, press materials, Khaki.pl. Watch: Coeur De Lion, press materials, Khaki.pl. Other images: Unsplash.com, Pixabay.com.

p. 84-85: Dresses, coat, and bag: Molton, press materials, Khaki.pl. Watch and earrings: Coeur De Lion, press materials, Khaki.pl. Other images: Pixabay.com.

p. 88-89: Clothing packshots, bag, and belt: Molton, press materials, Khaki.pl. Boots: Ochnik, press materials, Tweed.pl. Other images: Unsplash.com, Pixabay.com.

p. 100-101: Clothing packshots: Molton, press materials, Khaki.pl. Hat, shoes and other images: Unsplash.com, Pixabay.com.

p. 106-107: Clothing packshots and bag: Molton, press materials, Khaki.pl. Necklace: Ti Sento, press materials, Khaki.pl. Other images: Unsplash.com, Pixabay.com.

p. 110-111: Clothing packshots and bag: Molton, press materials, Khaki.pl. Other images: Unsplash.com, Pixabay.com.

p. 142-143: Clothing packshots: Molton, press materials, Khaki.pl. Other images: Unsplash.com, Pixabay.com.

p. 150-151: Clothing packshots, belt, and bag: Molton, press materials, Khaki.pl. Shoes: Ochnik, press materials, Tweed.pl. Other images: Unsplash.com, Pixabay.com.

p. 156-157: Clothing packshots and bag: Molton, press materials, Khaki.pl. Earrings: Nomination Italy, press materials, Khaki.pl. Other images: Unsplash.com, Pixabay.com.

p. 162-163: Clothing packshots: Molton, press materials, Khaki.pl. Earrings: Coeur De Lion, press materials, Khaki.pl. Other images: Unsplash.com, Pixabay.com.

All Moodboards by Laura Merano, © 2024.

Other Books by Laura Merano

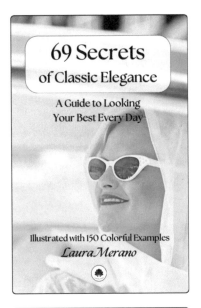

69 Secrets
of Classic Elegance

A Guide to Looking
Your Best Every Day

Illustrated with 150 Colorful Examples
Laura Merano

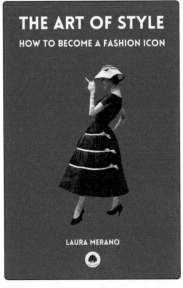

THE ART OF STYLE
HOW TO BECOME A FASHION ICON

LAURA MERANO

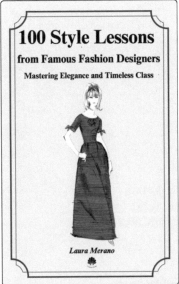

100 Style Lessons
from Famous Fashion Designers

Mastering Elegance and Timeless Class

Laura Merano

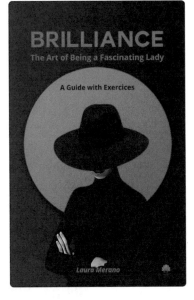

BRILLIANCE
The Art of Being a Fascinating Lady

A Guide with Exercices

Laura Merano

Coquille Dorée

Made in the USA
Columbia, SC
29 December 2024